Diagnosis and Treatment of Bone Tumors: A Team Approach

(A MAYO CLINIC MONOGRAPH)

Diagnosis and Treatment of Bone Tumors: A Team Approach

(A MAYO CLINIC MONOGRAPH)

Franklin H. Sim, M.D., Editor

ISBN No. 10-943432-01-4

Library of Congress No. 82-062397

To the many young people who
are victims of bone sarcoma;
may the courage they show in
their fight against this dreaded
tumor provide the energy for
continued research to find an
effective cure.

CONTENTS

CONTRIBUTORS

JOHN W. BEABOUT, M.D.
Consultant, Department of Diagnostic Radiology;* Associate Professor of Radiology†

WILLIAM E. BOWMAN, JR., M.D.
Resident in Orthopedics, Mayo Graduate School of Medicine, Rochester, Minnesota.

EDMUND Y. S. CHAO, Ph.D.
Consultant, Department of Orthopedics (Biomechanical Research);* Professor of Bioengineering†

KAY L. COOPER, M.D.
Consultant, Department of Diagnostic Radiology;* Assistant Professor of Radiology†

DAVID C. DAHLIN, M.D.
Consultant, Department of Pathology (Surgical Pathology);* Professor of Pathology†

JOHN H. EDMONSON, M.D.
Consultant, Department of Oncology (Medical Oncology);* Associate Professor of Oncology†

GERALD S. GILCHRIST, M.B., B.CH.
Consultant, Departments of Pediatrics and Internal Medicine (Hematology);* Professor of Pediatrics†

ALVARO MARTINEZ, M.D.
Consultant, Department of Oncology (Therapeutic Radiology);* Assistant Professor of Oncology†

RICHARD A. McLEOD, M.D.
Consultant, Department of Diagnostic Radiology;* Associate Professor of Radiology†

PETER C. PAIROLERO, M.D.
Consultant, Department of Surgery;* Associate Professor of Surgery†

DOUGLAS J. PRITCHARD, M.D.
Consultant, Department of Orthopedics;* Associate Professor of Orthopedic Surgery†

THOMAS C. SHIVES, M.D.
Consultant, Department of Orthopedics;* Assistant Professor of Orthopedic Surgery†

FRANKLIN H. SIM, M.D.
Consultant, Department of Orthopedics;* Associate Professor of Orthopedic Surgery†

HENRY H. STONNINGTON, M.B., B.S., M.S., F.R.C.P. (EDIN)
Consultant, Department of Physical Medicine and Rehabilitation;* Associate Professor of Physical Medicine and Rehabilitation†

ROBERT L. TELANDER, M.D.
Consultant, Department of Surgery (Pediatric Surgery);* Associate Professor of Surgery†

KRISHNAN K. UNNI, M.B., B.S.
Consultant, Department of Pathology (Surgical Pathology);* Associate Professor of Pathology†

LESTER E. WOLD, M.D.
Consultant, Department of Pathology (Surgical Pathology);* Instructor in Pathology†

*Mayo Clinic and Mayo Foundation, Rochester, Minnesota.
†Mayo Medical School, Rochester, Minnesota.

Foreword

"One of the strongest convictions of the Doctors Mayo was that the combined wisdom of a man's peers is greater than that of any individual" (1). It was probably not clairvoyance as much as common sense that led to this "team" approach to medical problems.

By the early 1900's, the father, William Worrall Mayo, had retired and the sons, Dr. William and Dr. Charles, were managing a very busy practice and, in addition, they were supervising the education of "associates" who were coming to Rochester in ever-increasing numbers for postgraduate training, especially in surgery.

It was clear by this time that there were to be surgeons, and nonsurgeons, later to be called internists—the cleavage between medicine and surgery had occurred—and there was no question but that Dr. Will and Dr. Charlie were to be surgeons.

Medical knowledge had begun to accumulate at an ever-quickening pace, and beyond the division of medical practice into medicine and surgery, the Mayos saw the need to bring specialization into surgery to better serve the patient. Such narrowing of surgical practice into special fields had already been started in the eastern United States and in England. Young associates were selected and sent away for the special training needed to establish departments of neurosurgery, orthopedics, urology, and, in time, many others as well.

This separation of surgical practice and training into special fields of endeavor worked quite well for a while. However, the territorial boundaries, as originally conceived, had to be redrawn as specialty boards and certification emerged in the years after World War II. The importance of the conflicts over who was to do what was overwhelmed by what had become an explosion of medical and general scientific knowledge. Not only was the "general surgeon" as a breed to become extinct (2), but the "generalist" in the several specialties seems en route to the same fate, for things are now so complex that no one person can "do it all." Subspecialization has become a fact of life, a required response to an undeniable need bearing precisely on the need to afford the patient the best possible care.

The Orthopedic Department of the Mayo Clinic responded to this need early by providing a Section of Hand Surgery soon after World War II. In the years that followed, other special sections devoted to pediatrics, adult reconstruction, trauma, microvascular surgery, and oncology were established, and, in addition, research laboratories in oncology and bioengineering were provided.

Under the provision of the National Cancer Act, Mayo Clinic was designated a Comprehensive Cancer Center in 1973, some 4 years after a Section of Surgical Oncology had started functioning in the Orthopedic Department. Already underway, and to be intensified later, were randomized prospective therapeutic trials (notably for cutaneous melanoma and for osteosarcoma), and, in addition, investigations were under way in basic oncologic research with emphasis on virology and immunology.

Just as the orthopedic generalist soon proved unable to serve adequately the needs of the tumor patient, neither could the surgical oncologist. The need for a multidisciplinary team approach was evident, and vital to the surgeon's work was the input from many specialties—the medical oncologist, the surgical pathologist, and the orthopedic radiologist. This multidisciplinary "team approach" now characterizes the Mayo Clinic practice and has been strengthened by the services of fields of expertise such as therapeutic radiology, rehabilitation service, and bioengineering.

Thus, the cancer patient (most of whom are now referred to designated centers) is getting better care. However, few of the major cancer problems have been solved in spite of this effort. The most pressing need, of course, is to find the etiologic agent (or agents) that cause musculoskeletal tumors. Presently, at least, the search has been elusive.

Meanwhile, while the search for an etiologic agent continues, treatment practices must be improved to increase effectiveness with regard to cure, and to reduce morbidity. Much of this effort demands prospective randomized trials and multi-institutional cooperation in these studies so that answers may be obtained more quickly. The organization of special interest groups, like the Musculoskeletal Tumor Society, creating a forum for discussion of mutual problems, does much to further this aim. Work now under way to develop reliable limb-salvage regimens typifies the problems that can be managed only in a center where multidisciplinary support is the routine, and whose final value can best be assessed by multi-institutional cooperation.

This volume, created by several members of the Mayo "team," is intended to picture the multidisciplinary approach at work, with the full realization and hope that the medicines and techniques now in use will soon be supplanted by something better.

John C. Ivins, M.D.

References

1. Harwick HJ: Forty-Four Years With the Mayo Clinic: 1908–1952. Rochester, Minnesota, Whiting Press, 1957
2. Smith GW: What is General Surgery? Who is a General Surgeon? (editorial) Arch Surg 116:853, 1981

Preface

While there are many varieties of bone tumors, primary
lesions of bone are relatively rare. These lesions may
confront the physician with many problems in recognition and
diagnosis. Although many advances have been made in
recent years in adjuvant treatment and reconstructive
surgery, close adherence to the well-established principles in
the evaluation of these tumors, as outlined in Chapter 3, is
essential. Musculoskeletal oncology demands high-quality
teamwork in order to assure effective management. Pitfalls
can be avoided and the results of treatment improved by the
coordination of the practitioner, orthopedic surgeon,
roentgenologist, and pathologist. This teamwork also involves
members of other disciplines, such as the radiotherapist,
medical oncologist, thoracic surgeon, rehabilitation specialist,
and bioengineer. In the management of bone tumors there
has been a trend toward the use of regional centers, where an
experienced bone pathologist is available and the cooperative
talents of these many disciplines can be utilized. This
cooperation not only facilitates the effective use of existing
technology but also allows other methods of investigation and
treatment of primary bone tumors to be explored and
evaluated.

This monograph emphasizes the multidisciplinary team
approach to the diagnosis and treatment of bone tumors
which is employed on a daily basis at the Mayo Clinic. This
approach is reflected in the multiple authorship by various
disciplines in most of the chapters. While not intended to be
all-encompassing, the monograph stresses the principles of
diagnosis and treatment of these challenging tumors.

Franklin H. Sim, M.D.

Diagnosis and Treatment of Bone Tumors: A Team Approach

(A MAYO CLINIC MONOGRAPH)

Section I:

General Information

CHAPTER 1

PATHOLOGY AND CLASSIFICATION

Lester E. Wold, M.D.
Krishnan K. Unni, M.B., B.S.
David C. Dahlin, M.D.

The treatment of orthopedic diseases has changed significantly during the last three decades. This change is particularly true of the therapeutic modalities employed for bone tumors. Resection of certain malignant tumors and the introduction of new chemotherapeutic and radiotherapeutic methods and protocols emphasize the need for accurate classification of bone tumors.

Pathology

The histologic appearance of bony lesions should be correlated with the radiographic appearance and the clinical setting in order to arrive at an accurate diagnosis. In this manner, the pathologist may have the differential diagnostic possibilities in mind before studying the biopsy material.

The radiographic appearance and clinical setting are also helpful in determining the type of biopsy procedure to be used. Schajowicz and Derqui (1) have advocated aspiration needle biopsy, particularly for vertebral lesions. Needle biopsy also can be used for spinal lesions; if the results are negative, an open biopsy follows. In this way, both the cytologic preparations and the material for paraffin embedding can be obtained. We have utilized open biopsy almost exclusively to obtain tissue. The most significant problem with respect to needle biopsy is the adequate sampling of the tumor. If the radiographic appearance of the lesion is suggestive of a malignant tumor, a negative needle biopsy is of no help. We believe that open biopsy is a more reliable method for obtaining a representative sample of the lesion.

Some specialized equipment is needed to process the biopsy specimens of bony lesions. Most bony tumors have soft parts. These parts either may be cut for frozen section or may be embedded in paraffin and cut without being decalcified. Even with sclerotic lesions, soft tissue often can be teased from between bony trabeculae using a needle or the tip of a scalpel blade. Specimens that require decalcification may be processed in various ways. We utilize 20% formic acid in 10% buffered formalin in our laboratory. This allows the specimen to be fixed while it is being decalcified. The specimen remains in this solution for 24 to 36 hours. After that time, it is washed in water for 2 to 3 hours. The tissue is then processed in the usual manner. Hydrochloric acid or nitric acid also may be used for decalcification. The tissue blocks must be cut thin (5-mm thick) to ensure rapid decalcification and to avoid artifacts from prolonged exposure to acid solutions.

Frozen sections are extremely helpful in the diagnosis and therapy of bony lesions. A final diagnosis often can be made on the basis of the frozen section of the soft portion of a tumor. When diagnosis is not possible, the adequacy of the biopsy material can be evaluated. Such evaluation is extremely important, as one of the major sources of error in open biopsy is inadequacy of the tissue for diagnosis—for example, a specimen from the edge of a lesion may show only reactive new bone formation. In addition, frozen sections can be used to identify lesions that are inflammatory and therefore should be cultured. The nature of the inflammatory infiltrate will help in suggesting the cause and the type of culture medium that should be employed, for example, bacterial versus fungal or tuberculous. Finally, frozen sections should be used to check the margins of resection for involvement with tumor. Various stains may be used in staining frozen sections. In our laboratory, we use methylene blue. However, in evaluating cartilagenous lesions, staining with hematoxylin is often helpful in obtaining better cytologic definition. Tissue that is approximately 10 μm in thickness can be fixed 1 minute before staining with hematoxylin, which requires approximately 1 more minute.

When amputation, disarticulation, or resection is done, the margin of the specimen should be examined to determine the adequacy of the resection. The soft tissues then should be carefully dissected from the bone. With the specimen held in a bench vise, the bone can be cut with a band saw or a butcher's meat saw. Small bones or bony lesions can be more easily cut with a jig saw. Thin sections (5 to 10 mm) can be obtained in this manner if radiography of the specimen is desired. The cut surface of the bone should be washed to remove "bone dust," and the dimensions of the tumor and its relationship to the surface and margins of resection should be recorded. Samples of the soft portions may be cut immediately for frozen section or embedding. Areas that appear to be grossly different should be

Table 1-1. Classification of Bone Tumors

Histologic type	Benign	Malignant
Hematopoietic	. . .	Myeloma
		Lymphoma
Chondrogenic	Osteochondroma	Chondrosarcoma and variants
	Chondroma	
	Chondroblastoma	
	Chondromyxoid fibroma	
Osteogenic	Osteoid osteoma	Osteosarcoma and variants
	Osteoblastoma	
Unknown origin	Giant cell tumor	Malignant giant cell tumor
	(?)Fibrous histiocytoma	Ewing's tumor
		Adamantinoma
		(?)Malignant fibrous histiocytoma
Fibrogenic	Desmoplastic fibroma	Fibrosarcoma
Notochordal	. . .	Chordoma
Vascular	Hemangioma	Hemangioendotheliosarcoma
		Hemangiopericytoma

sampled and submitted for permanent section. The soft tissues should be examined for lymph nodal or vascular involvement. If frozen sections reveal that the tumor is a small-cell malignant neoplasm, it may be helpful to fix a piece of tissue in 80% alcohol for subsequent periodic acid-Schiff staining.

Radiography of the specimen is of limited usefulness in diagnosis, except in cases of osteoid osteoma. In these cases, specimen radiography of the bony fragments removed at operation may reveal a rarefied or sclerotic nidus. Specimen radiography also may reveal an infarct or enchondroma associated with a malignancy. However, careful gross analysis can do as well. Imprint techniques may be useful in the differential diagnosis of small round-cell tumors, but good-quality frozen and permanent sections fulfill the same purpose. Finally, electron microscopy is still of limited usefulness in diagnostic bone pathology.

Classification

The classification of bone tumors is based upon the cytology of the tumor cells or the matrix they produce (or both). The classification originally proposed by Lichtenstein (2) is generally used, with minor modifications (Table 1-1).

References

1. Schajowicz F, Derqui JC: Puncture biopsy in lesions of the locomotor system: review of results of 4050 cases, including 941 vertebral punctures. Cancer 21:531–548, 1968
2. Lichtenstein L: Classification of primary tumors of bone. Cancer 4:335–341, 1951

CHAPTER 2

RADIOLOGIC EVALUATION

Kay L. Cooper, M.D.
Richard A. McLeod, M.D.
John W. Beabout, M.D.

Many sophisticated imaging techniques for the diagnosis of disease are now available to the radiologist. For the radiologic diagnosis of bone tumors, however, routine radiographs remain the most informative and essential diagnostic modality. Routine plain films most accurately display the type of bone destruction and the nature of the margin between tumor and normal bone. The extent and type of periosteal new bone and of tumor matrix mineralization are well visualized on plain films. In many instances, a specific diagnosis can be suggested on the basis of the radiographic findings, and no additional diagnostic studies are indicated.

Conventional tomography may help to localize or more completely visualize certain tumors. An excellent example is osteoid osteoma. Tomograms can accurately locate the small lucent nidus within an area of dense cortical thickening or within complex structures such as the vertebral neural arch (Fig. 2-1). By eliminating superimposed structures, tomography can display subtle details of the tumor that might not otherwise be appreciated. The tumor margins, internal mineralization, and pathologic fractures are all well demonstrated with tomography.

In nearly all instances, computed tomography (CT) is less useful than plain films in identifying the tumor and arriving at a specific diagnosis. Exceptions occur in complex anatomic areas such as the spinal column and sacrum. CT may detect lesions in these areas which were not appreciated on plain films. CT scans in patients with multiple myeloma may show innumerable tiny lytic areas, while routine radiographs and isotope bone scans show no abnormalities. The major contribution of CT is in determining the extent of the process, especially the extent of the associated soft-tissue component. CT generally adds useful information about tumor extent and is almost invariably helpful when the lesion is in the central skeleton (Fig. 2-2). CT is less useful in evaluating peripheral lesions, but it can be helpful in determining if a limb-salvage procedure is possible (1). CT is also useful in some cases in demonstrating tumor extent in the medullary canal as well as in accurately depicting tumor density, composition, and mineralization (2). In the preoperative staging and follow-up of malignant bone tumors, CT scans of the chest have proved invaluable in the detection of metastatic lesions of the lung.

In the past, angiography had only a very minor role in the evaluation of primary bone tumors. With the advent of CT, this role has become almost nonexistent. The extent of the tumor and the major vascular relationships are well demonstrated by CT.

Another major imaging modality is the isotope bone scan. Because of its nonspecificity, this procedure is more useful in the detection or exclusion of additional lesions than in the characterization of individual lesions. In some cases, the extent of the tumor is better demonstrated on nuclear scans.

The impression gained from the initial radiograph will de-

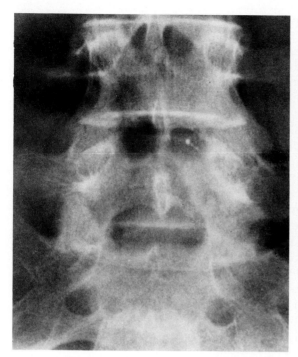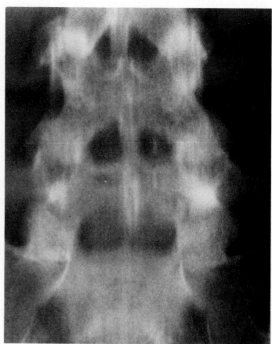

Fig. 2-1.

Fig. 2-1. Value of tomography in demonstrating an osteoid osteoma. Small calcified nidus in left lamina of L-5 is much more apparent on tomogram (B) than on plain film (A).

Fig. 2-2. *A*, Radiograph of sacrum shows abnormal lucency in lower sacrum. Detail is obscured by overlapping bowel content. *B*, CT scan shows sacral destruction by the chordoma and a soft tissue mass extending anteriorly.

termine which additional studies are necessary. Benign lesions demonstrate such radiographic features as sharp margination, expansion, intact cortex, and smooth, uniform periosteal new bone. In these cases, other diagnostic studies are seldom necessary. Occasionally, tomography demonstrates additional findings, clarifying the diagnosis. If surgery is indicated, patients will then proceed directly to biopsy.

Plain-film findings of cortical breakthrough, poor margination, permeative destruction, irregular or spiculated periosteal new bone, and tumor new bone formation are indicative of a malignant bone tumor. In these cases, the diagnostic workup is generally more extensive. Tomograms may be used to improve visualization of fine detail. Isotope bone scans help define tumor extent and exclude or detect additional lesions. CT is often done, especially in cases of central lesions or in peripheral lesions if limb salvage is contemplated. This is usually done in conjunction with CT scan of the lungs in search of pulmonary metastatic disease. Biopsy and the appropriate surgery are then indicated.

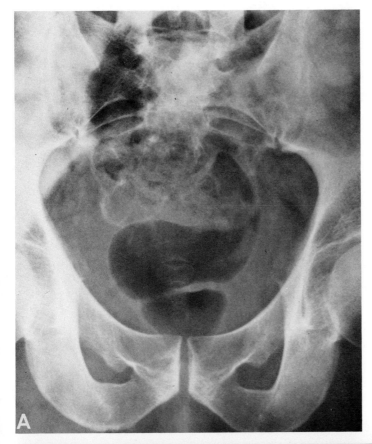

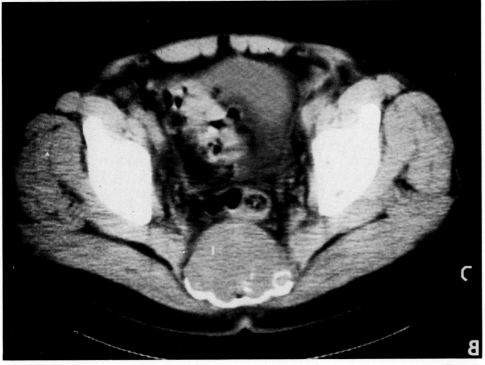

Fig. 2-2.

To arrive at the correct diagnosis, the radiologist needs to correlate information derived from these roentgenographic studies with the clinical findings and often, ultimately, with the pathologic findings. The specific radiologic features of each osseous lesion and the clinicopathologic correlation are outlined in the respective chapters.

References

1. Lukens JA, McLeod RA, Sim FH: Computed tomographic evaluation of primary osseous malignant neoplasms. AJR 139:45–48, 1982
2. McLeod RA, Stephens DH, Beabout JW, et al: Computed tomography of the skeletal system. Semin Roentgenol 13:235–247, 1978

Chapter 3

CLINICAL EVALUATION

Douglas J. Pritchard, M.D.

The clinical evaluation of the patient with a bone tumor may be divided into three phases. First is the discovery phase, in which the bone lesion is found; second is the prebiopsy diagnostic phase, in which all of the relevant diagnoses are considered; and third is the prebiopsy planning phase, in which all preoperative evaluations may be accomplished.

Discovery Phase

One of the difficulties in the diagnosis of bone tumors is their rarity. Few physicians encounter enough bone tumors in their practice to be comfortable with the diagnosis. Most physicians, however, are able to assess the patient and to find the lesion. It is not uncommon for a patient to have experienced an injury at the site of a previously unsuspected tumor and then to seek medical attention because of the injury. It is probably axiomatic that if the patient is sufficiently symptomatic from an injury to seek medical attention, then the site in question should be examined. This is particularly necessary when the symptoms seem out of proportion to the extent of the injury. Occasionally, a bone tumor may remain asymptomatic until fracture occurs through the lesion. Thus, when a fracture develops from trivial or minimal injury, the presence of a pathologic fracture should be suspected.

One of the problems in finding bone tumors is that the pain may be referred to a site remote from the actual tumor. This is particularly true with lesions in the region of the hip joint, where they tend to cause referred knee pain. Another problem is that while a tumor may be present within bone, it may not be readily visualized even with good-quality roentgenograms. For example, a chondrosarcoma may arise on the inner wall of the acetabulum in an adult and yet may not be visible on roentgenograms of the hip. If the patient also has degenerative joint disease, the problem is compounded because this common problem is readily detectable, whereas the subtle findings of chondrosarcoma may not be appreciated. Osteoid osteoma is another tumor that is difficult to visualize on roentgenograms. This lesion tends to produce referred pain and localized atrophy—features that may confuse the physician. In addition, when osteoid osteoma occurs in the region of the spinal column, scoliosis may be present. Thus, it is necessary to have a high index of suspicion. Although bone tumors are, in general, rare, when they occur, they may have a devastating effect on the patient.

Diagnostic Phase

Once a bone lesion has been found, the next problem is to decide what the diagnostic possibilities are. A reasonable differential diagnosis can be established based on the roentgenographic appearance of the lesion and the clinical information. However, other conditions besides tumors may affect bone, some of which may simulate bone tumors. It is helpful to have a number of diagnoses in mind so that they can be ruled out. Trauma can cause lesions in bone. A stress fracture, for example, may simulate a bone tumor. Healing avulsion fractures may cause a mass that simulates a tumor. Infections may mimic almost any of the bone tumors: osteomyelitis is particularly likely to be confused with Ewing's sarcoma. Certain metabolic bone conditions may be associated with bone lesions. For example, the so-called brown tumor of hyperparathyroidism is similar roentgenographically and histologically to benign giant cell tumor of bone. Certain circulatory disorders may cause bone lesions. For example, an infarct may be confused with a chondrosarcoma. Synovial disease may cause bone lesions—for example, the cysts that are associated with pigmented villonodular synovitis. All these possibilities should be considered in the differential diagnosis.

The patient's medical history may be of some help. The patient usually complains of pain of varying duration. The onset of pain may be very gradual, or the pain may begin when a pathologic fracture occurs through a fairly extensive tumor. Night pain, especially if it is relieved by salicylates, is characteristic of osteoid osteoma. Otherwise the character of the pain is rather nonspecific. Occasionally, the patient has a mass as the first symptom. The mass is likely to be a soft-tissue extension of a primary bone tumor or an osteochondroma or a growth from the surface of the bone.

The patient's age is very helpful in the differential diagnosis. Certain conditions are likely to have their onset at certain ages. For example, more than 80% of benign giant cell tumors occur in patients who are at least 20 years old, whereas more than 80% of aneurysmal bone cysts and chondroblastomas, with which giant cell tumors may be confused, occur in patients who are less than 20 years old. Chondrosarcoma tends to occur in older adults, whereas osteosarcoma tends to develop in teenagers. Neuroblastoma metastatic to bone occurs in infants, whereas Ewing's sarcoma occurs in older children.

The patient's sex is less helpful in that nearly all of the bone tumors are more common in males than in females, with the exception of benign giant cell tumor of bone. The tendency, however, is not sufficiently strong to be of much practical help.

The site of the lesion is important in that certain tumors have a predilection for certain bones or certain locations within a bone. For example, osteosarcoma tends to occur in the distal femur and usually arises in the metaphyseal region of the femur. Enchondroma tends to occur in the small bones of the hands and feet, but it may also occur in other bones. Both chondroblastoma and giant cell tumor tend to arise in the epiphysis. Hence, the location of the tumor provides valuable diagnostic information. Other factors in the patient's history are unlikely to be of much help in the differential diagnosis. The family history may, on occasion, be helpful—for example, in the case of multiple osteochondromas. Finally, a history of exposure to various toxic agents or to prior radiation may be of diagnostic importance.

The physical examination is of limited help in the differential diagnosis. Practically all bone tumors may on occasion produce a palpable mass. Increased warmth and dilated veins may be noted over the mass, particularly with malignant tumors. These findings are so nonspecific, however, as to be of minimal value.

Although many other diagnostic measures may be taken, plain roentgenograms provide the basis for a differential diagnosis, particularly when combined with knowledge of the patient's age and other information, as previously discussed. Once it is decided that the patient may have a bone tumor, it must be borne in mind that metastatic lesions are much more common than primary bone tumors and that primary bone tumors may be either benign or malignant. In addition, of the primary malignant bone tumors, some are radioresistant and some are radiosensitive. Once an initial assessment has been made, various decisions can be made. It is helpful to approach the diagnostic phase as a team effort, taking into consideration the expertise of a diagnostic radiologist with a particular interest in bone tumors. At this stage, certain patients may be observed without the need for a biopsy—for example, the patient who presents with a small osteochondroma that is relatively asymptomatic. Similarly, if there is convincing roentgenographic and clinical evidence suggesting that the patient has a stress fracture, then biopsy is not necessary. It may be that, at this point in the evaluation, more information is needed. In addition to the plain roentgenograms, a tomogram may be useful in demonstrating more clearly the characteristics of the tumor, as well as in helping to delineate the extent of the tumor. Computed tomography (CT) is also very helpful in this regard. Although not providing much information about the actual diagnosis, CT gives a more accurate assessment of the extent of the lesion and may actually help with the diagnosis. For example, a circumferential tumor surrounding a long bone may appear to involve the medullary canal on plain roentgenograms and even on linear tomography, but cross-sections obtained on CT may show that the lesion is parosteal and not intermedullary. If the radiographic features are otherwise compatible with the diagnosis of an osteosarcoma, in this situation the diagnosis would be a parosteal osteosarcoma.

At this time, information about the potential usefulness of the nuclear magnetic resonator as a diagnostic modality is scarce, but it may prove to be useful. Bone scans, whether technetium-99 or gallium, rarely offer much diagnostic information, but occasionally they are helpful. For example, if an older patient has a destructive lesion and the bone scan is negative at the site of the suspected tumor, the diagnosis is likely myeloma. However, for most tumors the bone scan is useful only insofar as it helps determine the extent of the disease. My colleagues and I do not routinely employ angiography in the assessment of bone tumors, although other institutions do. If it is necessary to determine the location of the major vessels in relation to the tumor, then contrast medium can be used with CT. This allows information to be obtained by a noninvasive method rather than by invasive conventional angiography. We are not impressed with the usefulness of angiography in the differential diagnosis.

Conventional laboratory studies occasionally may also be useful. For example, if there is a destructive lesion in the end of the femur, the serum calcium level should be measured to rule out the possibility of hyperparathyroidism. Similarly, the patient with Ewing's sarcoma may have mild leukocytosis or anemia or both. A growing neoplasm may cause an elevation of the serum alkaline phosphatase level. The value of an elevated alkaline phosphatase is difficult to assess in children, but it may have some importance in the adult.

Preoperative Phase

Once the lesion has been found and a diagnosis has been made, the preoperative planning may proceed. As previously mentioned, surgery is not indicated in some situations. However, if it is clear that a biopsy is needed and that subsequent surgery may be necessary, depending upon the results of the biopsy, then further planning is necessary. The major considerations are the location, extent, and nature of the tumor. The various diagnostic modalities utilized in the differential diagnosis also provide useful information about the location and extent of the lesion, and the results of biopsy should supply data on the nature of the lesion. Each case must be individualized. If, for example, a lesion has roentgenographic and clinical features suggestive of a primary malignant bone tumor, one should try to rule out systemic metastatic disease. In this regard, a technetium bone scan may be useful, and CT of the lung fields may reveal occult metastatic disease that is not visible on plain roentgenograms of the chest. This information should be obtained before the biopsy specimen is taken because, if the tumor does prove to be malignant and CT is required, CT should be done before the patient is subjected to a general anesthetic since postoperative atelectasis or minor changes that will confuse the situation may develop after the operation. In addition, it is better to have information about the presence of metastatic disease before a definitive decision is made regarding the extent of surgery. For tumors that appear to arise from the bones of the pelvis, CT of the pelvis is very useful, although excretory urography, barium enema study, or proctoscopic examination may be necessary before the bone biopsy specimen is taken.

Summary

The stepwise but individualized evaluation of the patient with a known or suspected bone tumor allows one to avoid some of the common pitfalls that may otherwise jeopardize the patient's management. The team approach utilizing the clinician, radiologist, and pathologist is the best assurance that many potential problems will be avoided. Management of specific tumor entities will be discussed in other chapters.

CHAPTER 4

PRINCIPLES OF SURGICAL TREATMENT

Franklin H. Sim, M.D.

After discovery of an osseous lesion, the decision as to the most effective treatment demands thorough clinical, roentgenographic, and pathologic evaluations. Treatment is based on an accurate histologic diagnosis, and this requires an adequate biopsy specimen. Preoperative clinical staging varies with the nature of the tumor. If the lesion appears to be typically benign, a relatively limited set of examinations may be indicated. If, however, the lesion appears to be malignant, more extensive preoperative evaluation is necessary. In the latter instance, the pretreatment assessment must determine the patient's general health and whether there is evidence of occult or systemic metastasis. The specialized studies necessary to determine the regional extent of involvement of the tumor are outlined in the chapter on clinical evaluation (Chapter 3). An extensive evaluation is usually necessary in making the therapeutic decision, particularly to determine whether a limb-saving resection can be performed or amputation is preferred.

Biopsy

Careful preoperative planning and removal of the biopsy specimen are extremely important. Because the histologic interpretation of these tumors is difficult, it is necessary to provide the pathologist with an adequate sample of representative tissue for study. There are instances in which needle biopsy may be useful (1)—for example, when the patient has a known primary adenocarcinoma and biopsy has been done to confirm metastatic disease. Lesions metastatic to the spinal column are probably the most common lesions in which needle biopsy is used. Close rapport between the pathologist and the surgeon is necessary when utilizing this technique (2). In general, however, particularly in primary tumors, needle biopsy does not provide enough representative tissue to meet the requirements of the surgical pathologist.

In these cases, an open biopsy procedure must be planned, with a definitive surgical procedure in mind. The incision should be as small as possible and placed where it will not compromise the definitive surgical procedure. For example, when amputation is anticipated, the biopsy incision must be performed at a site that will not interfere with the amputation flaps (Fig. 4-1). If a resection is performed, the location of the biopsy site is critical since the site must be removed en bloc with the tumor; thus, if the entire distal end of the femur is to be resected, in which case a medial incision is usually preferred, the biopsy incision should be made in line with the proposed definitive incision so that the entire biopsy tract can be included in the resection. A poorly planned biopsy incision would make the en bloc resection unsuccessful if the definitive surgery is unable to remove the biopsy-contaminated tissue. For example, when a biopsy of the upper part of the humerus contaminates the neurovascular area, a limb-saving Tinkoff-Lindberg resection will not

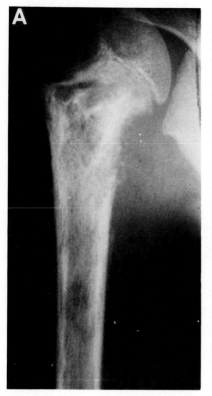

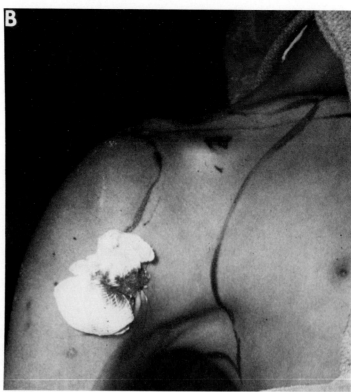

Fig. 4-1. *A*, Anteroposterior view of shoulder showing osteosarcoma of proximal humerus. *B*, Biopsy site over the proximal humerus, distant from the amputation flap.

be effective, and a forequarter amputation will be required. Moreover, the possibility of future radiation treatment must be considered when planning a biopsy so that the area can easily be included in the field of radiation.

A transverse wound on an extremity should be avoided because this makes definitive surgery particularly difficult. With bone tumors, the biopsy incision should be placed directly over a muscle belly, and the muscle rather than the plane between the muscles should be transected. In this way, the amount of soft-tissue dissection is minimized and the muscle tissue can be closed over the biopsy site. This approach reduces the chances of the tumor's spreading along fascial planes. If the tumor extends through cortical bone and into adjacent soft tissues, a biopsy specimen of this tissue should be taken rather than the bone itself being entered. This approach will provide adequate tissue and also minimize the chances of subsequent pathologic fractures at the biopsy site in a radioresponsive tumor. If the cortex of the bone must be windowed, from the biomechanical standpoint, the defect should be made small and round and placed at the least mechanically stressed site in order to avoid the potential of a pathologic fracture, particularly in a weight-bearing bone. Hemostasis is essential. Plugging the biopsy window with gel foam or methyl methacrylate is effective. The biopsy wound should be carefully closed to minimize hematoma formation and soft-tissue seating.

Great care must be exerted when taking a biopsy specimen of cartilage lesions because of the high potential for seeding of the soft tissues, with subsequent implants and local recurrence. In cartilage lesions, where pathologic interpretation may be difficult, an incisional biopsy specimen may not be representative, and an initial excision of the cartilage lesion may be advantageous, depending on its location and size. Excisional biopsy may be more readily performed in lesions of the pelvis.

Previously, my colleagues and I utilized a sterile tourniquet placed proximal to the tumor in an effort to avoid further dissemination of tumor cells into the bloodstream during the taking of the biopsy specimen (3). However, there has been no evidence to suggest that this has improved survival of patients with malignant tumors, and this technique has been abandoned (4). In addition to the alteration of the dynamics of the interosseous circulation by the tourniquet, as well as possible compression of an ill-defined soft-tissue mass, there are several theoretic reasons to discourage the use of the tourniquet. The demonstration of the consistency of circulating tumor cells, in addition to the demonstration of the role of fibrin clots in the implanting of metastatic deposits, suggests that the congestion distal to the tourniquet may have an adverse effect.

Clinical staging should be done before the biopsy procedure for two reasons. First, the findings in the studies (bone scan, computed tomographic scan, and angiography) that are necessary in planning treatment may be altered by the selection of the biopsy site (5). Second, the biopsy and definitive therapy should be done at the same time (4). Part of the tumor will contain soft tissue, which can be prepared by rapid frozen-section technique and analyzed by a pathologist who is experienced in histologic interpretation of malignant tumors of bone. This requires a laboratory equipped to do rapid frozen sectioning and an orthopedic surgeon who has competence in the pathologist's interpretation and in his own judgment and who can proceed with definitive therapy after the diagnosis has been made. Many surgical pathologists prefer to wait for permanent sections before they make a final diagnosis. This necessitates a delay between the taking of the biopsy specimen and the definitive procedure. While there is no conclusive evidence that a short delay affects the ultimate outcome, this delay should be kept as short as possible.

Treatment

Treatment is largely dictated by the natural history of the tumor. An adequate surgical procedure has been the most effective means of treating most patients who have primary radioresistant bone tumors. The objectives of surgical treatment are to remove the tumor completely and yet preserve as much function as possible without compromising the result. The surgical spectrum for the treatment of bone tumors includes simple biopsy, curettage with or without bone graft, excision, resection, ablative amputation, and even cryosurgery. Unfortunately, it is very difficult to review and compare retrospective experience or to evaluate prospective studies in the treatment of bone tumors because of the lack of a precise definition of the surgical procedure. Recently, progress has been made in developing a surgical staging system for both bone and soft-tissue sarcomas which can be correlated with the surgical procedure. In this system proposed by Enneking (6) (Table 4-1), three factors must be assessed: the surgical grade, the surgical site, and the presence of metastasis. Stage I indicates a low-grade lesion, and stage II a high-grade lesion. This reflects the biologic aggressiveness of the lesion and dictates the appropriate surgical margin. The stage is subdivided according to whether the tumor is intracompartmental (confined to the bone) or whether it erodes through the bone and has a subperiosteal or an extraosseous extension (Fig. 4-2). The presence of metastasis places the tumor in stage III (Table 4-1).

The surgical procedures are then described—first in terms of the surgical margin in relationship to the tumor and its surrounding reactive zone and second in terms of the technique in which these margins are accomplished (Fig. 4-3). In an intralesional margin, the plane of dissection violates the pseudocapsule, while a marginal margin has a narrow plane of dissection adjacent to the reactive pseudocapsule. A wide margin has a cuff of nonreactive normal tissue peripheral to all its margins, but the entire bone is not removed. By definition, a radical margin is achieved with removal of the entire bone. The surgical procedure can now be standardized and related to the surgical stage of the tumor.

In the recent proposal by Enneking and associates (6), the surgical procedures for bone tumors may be classified and stand-

Table 4-1. Surgical Staging of Bone Tumors

Stage	Grade	Site
IA	Low (G_1)	Intracompartmental (T_1)
IB	Low (G_1)	Extracompartmental (T_2)
IIA	High (G_2)	Intracompartmental (T_1)
IIB	High (G_2)	Extracompartmental (T_2)
III	Any (G) regional or distant metastasis	Any (T)

From Enneking WF, Spanier SS, Goodman MA: A system for the surgical staging of musculoskeletal sarcoma. Clin Orthop 153:106–120, 1980. By permission of JB Lippincott Company.

Bone Tumors

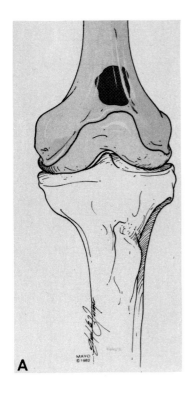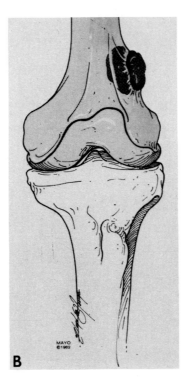

Fig. 4-2. *A*, Intracompartmental lesion (T_1) without extraosseous extension. *B*, Extracompartmental lesion (T_2) extending through cortex, with soft-tissue involvement.

ardized on a scale of 1 through 4 and related to the surgical stage of the lesion (Table 4-2). These margins may be achieved either by a local procedure or by amputation. For most low-grade lesions, treatment may be more conservative, while more radical procedures are necessary for the high-grade tumors. In this classification, grade 1 surgical treatment includes any procedure in which the plane of dissection violates the tumor or pseudocapsule. This includes intralesional curettage with or without the addition of physical agents. A grade 2 procedure corresponds to simple excision with a marginal margin around the lesion. A grade 3 procedure achieves a wide margin, and this can be accomplished by an en bloc excision or a cross-bone amputation. A grade 4 procedure corresponds to a radical resection in which the entire bone is removed, such as in a scapulectomy or a disarticulation.

Surgical Alternatives

Treatment is largely dictated by the nature of the lesion. Most benign and most low-grade malignant lesions may be managed with relatively conservative procedures, while high-grade lesions require more aggressive treatment.

Curettage. For benign bone tumors, the aims of controlling the disease and preserving function in the bone and neighboring joint can be achieved by curettage or simple excision; this would correspond to grade 1 or 2 surgical treatment in the classification

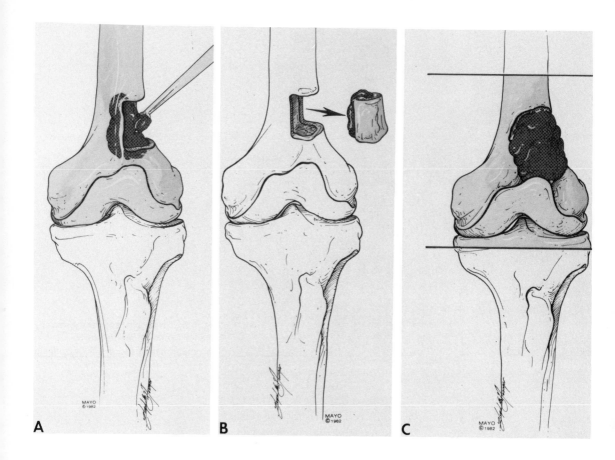

Fig. 4-3. *A*, Intralesional margin. *B*, Marginal margin. *C*, Wide margin.

Table 4-2. Grading System for Surgical Procedures in the Treatment of Bone Tumors

Grade	Margin	Local	Amputation
1	Intralesional	Curettage or debulking	Debulking or amputation
2	Marginal	Marginal excision	Marginal amputation
3	Wide	Wide local excision	Wide through-bone amputation
4	Radical	Radical local resection	Radical disarticulation

From Enneking WF, Spanier SS, Goodman MA: A system for the surgical staging of musculoskeletal sarcoma. Clin Orthop 153:106–120, 1980. By permission of JB Lippincott Company.

of Enneking. Treatment may need to be modified, depending on the surgical accessibility of the lesion or the presence of the lesion near the growth plate in a child. While certain measures must be taken if curettage is to be effective, probably the single most important factor is adequate exposure. Obtaining such

Bone Tumors

exposure requires making a large cortical window and completely exteriorizing the tumor cavity (Fig. 4-4). All aspects of the tumor cavity must be visualized. This may require removal of half or more of the circumference of the bone. Failure to exteriorize completely the tumor cavity with curettage through a small hole in the cortex routinely leads to recurrence (Fig. 4-4).

The tumor must be thoroughly excised with a sharp curette, followed by the use of a dental burr to extend the margin. After wide exteriorization and vigorous curettage, the soft tissues are packed with Vaseline gauze and moist sponges, and the curetted tumor cavity is filled with phenol for 30 to 45 seconds. Phenol,

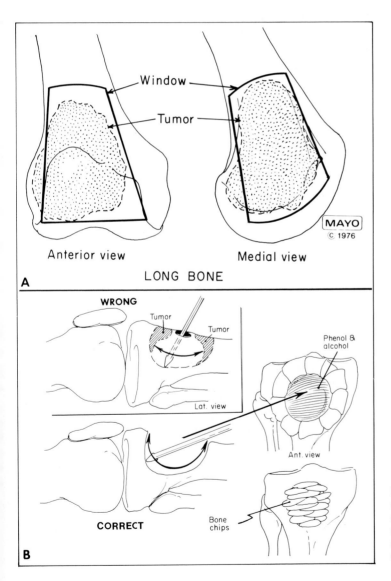

Fig. 4-4. *A*, Diagramatic illustration of wide exteriorization of lesion of distal femur, demonstrating an adequate excision by curettage. *B*, Diagramatic illustration showing the correct and the incorrect technique of curettage.

which coagulates protein, is effective in reaching the center of the cortical bone into which the tumor has permeated. The phenol is removed, and the cavity is rinsed with 95% acid alcohol. The curetted cavity is then lavaged vigorously with large amounts of isotonic saline (Fig. 4-4).

After curettage and chemical cautery, bone grafts are placed. Depending on the location and relationship to the joints, strut grafts may be necessary to support the articular surface. While reports in the literature indicate that there is a lower incidence of recurrence after curettage and bone grafting than after curettage alone, the grafts have no effect on recurrence of the tumor, but their need is indicative of a more radical and adequate excision. Methyl methacrylate also has been used effectively to fill these large defects after curettage. A variation of this procedure is excision curettage, which would be classified as a grade 1 surgical procedure. This procedure is more radical than simple curettage because either a marginal or a wide margin is achieved around most of the tumor, with the curettage being done in the subchondral region in an attempt to preserve the joint.

Resection. While conservative excision as the initial treatment is usually effective in most benign osseous lesions, aggressive and recurrent benign tumors require en bloc resection for eradication. For example, if initially a giant cell tumor is large and aggressive and has broken through the cortex, with soft-tissue extension (Campanacci [7] grade III), a complete resection is indicated. Occasionally, depending on location, a benign lesion may be resected, with preservation of the adjacent joint. However, since giant cell tumors are usually located in the end of the bone, wide excision, when indicated, will require removal of a large segment of the adjacent joint. This procedure necessitates a major reconstructive effort in order to restore function in the extremity. These techniques are outlined in Chapter 8, on limb salvage. Moreover, some malignant lesions lend themselves to effective treatment by wide excision, particularly low-grade chondrosarcoma, periosteal osteosarcoma, and other low-grade sarcomas.

In recent years, there has been increased interest in limb-saving radical en bloc resection for osteosarcoma and other high-grade radioresistant lesions (8-11). This is a valid alternative to amputation in carefully selected patients. The location and extent of the tumor must be favorable to enable removal with margins sufficient to prevent recurrence but not so extensive as to exclude restoration of useful function. Our criterion for resection of these lesions has been conservative—that is, for resection, the tumor should be largely interosseous and involve a reasonably short segment of the affected bone or, if there is extraosseous extension, the extension should be small and not involve neurovascular structures (Fig. 4-5). Also, at resection, if the tumor capsule is visualized or violated or if tumor cells spill into the wound and the wound becomes contaminated, it is best to proceed with amputation. Patient age is another consideration. Generally, the reconstructive techniques utilized after resection are applicable to older patients whose epiphyses have closed; for younger patients in childhood who are still growing, the expected limb-length discrepancy makes amputation the only realistic surgical procedure. Previous treatment and the stage of the disease may be other considerations. Additionally, there is recent interest in surgical resection of localized Ewing's sarcoma (12) in an attempt to improve local control and reduce morbidity in selected patients.

Amputation. At the present state of the art, for patients with high-grade aggressive tumors such as conventional osteosarcoma, when the lesion has invaded the surrounding soft tissues, an adequate margin can be achieved best by amputation. The level of amputation has been the source of continued debate. The first goal is to eradicate the tumor completely. The surgeon's second responsibility is to preserve as much function as possible. Experience has indicated that there is no added safety in leaving a joint between the tumor and the site of amputation (3), and my colleagues and I have traditionally done cross-bone amputation for low femoral lesions, striving to achieve a margin of 8 to 10 cm, as judged on the roentgenogram and bone scan (Fig. 4-6). Amputation at this level is preferred because of the better functional restoration and better quality of life that this affords the amputee, compared with disarticulation. At the time of amputation, the proximal marrow is checked by frozen-section analysis.

In large, extensive lesions or diaphyseal lesions, an adequate margin can be achieved best by disarticulation. Moreover, Enneking's documentation (13) of clinically undetectable intramedullary skip lesions separate from the primary lesion has encouraged some surgeons to prefer disarticulation when low femoral lesions are present. However, local recurrence has not been a clinical problem in our experience. In 100 consecutive cross-bone amputations, only two stump recurrences have been documented (4). However, if survival is prolonged by the use of chemotherapy, this could be a bigger clinical problem in the future.

Conclusion

Treatment must be based on an accurate histologic diagnosis. The removal of the biopsy specimen is extremely important, as a poorly placed biopsy incision may adversely affect the outcome of the definitive surgery. While there are many surgical options available, the decision as to the best method must be made after a thorough evaluation. The surgical staging system as proposed by Enneking is useful in individualizing the extent of the surgical procedure to the biologic aggressiveness of the tumor.

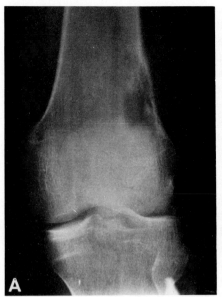
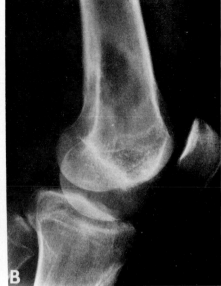
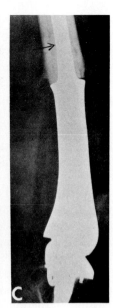

Fig. 4-5. Anteroposterior (*A*) and lateral (*B*) views of distal femur, showing osteosarcoma. This lesion met the criteria for limb-saving resection. *C*, After reconstruction with a custom total knee arthroplasty.

Fig. 4-6. Diagramatic illustration of level of amputation for resistant sarcoma of lower extremity.

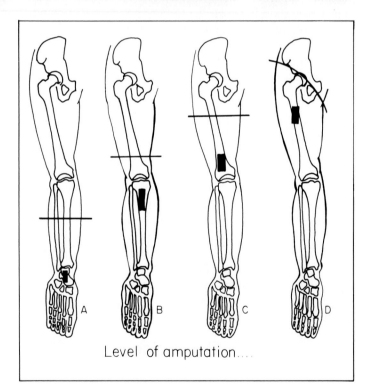

Level of amputation....

Fig. 4-6.

References

1. Craig FS: Metastatic and primary lesions of bone. Clin Orthop 73:33–38, 1970
2. Schajowicz F, Derqui JC: Puncture biopsy in lesions of the locomotor system: review of results in 4050 cases, including 941 vertebral punctures. Cancer 21:531–548, 1968
3. Dahlin DC, Coventry MB: Osteogenic sarcoma: a study of six hundred cases. J Bone Joint Surg [Am] 49:101–110, 1967
4. Sim FH, Ivins JC, Pritchard DJ: Surgical treatment of osteogenic sarcoma at the Mayo Clinic. Cancer Treat Rep 62:205–211, 1978
5. Enneking WF, Springfield DS: Osteosarcoma. Orthop Clin North Am 8:785–803, 1977
6. Enneking WF, Spanier SS, Goodman MA: A system for the surgical staging of musculoskeletal sarcoma. Clin Orthop 153:106–120, 1980
7. Campanacci M, Giunti A, Olmi R: Giant-cell tumours of bone: a study of 209 cases with long-term follow-up in 130. Ital J Orthop Traumatol 1:249–277, 1975
8. Johnston JO: Local resection in primary malignant bone tumors. Clin Orthop 153:73–80, 1980
9. Martin RG, Lindberg RD, Russell WO: Preoperative radiotherapy and surgery in the management of soft tissue sarcoma. *In* Management of Primary Bone and Soft Tissue Tumors. Chicago, Year Book Medical Publishers, 1977, pp 299–307
10. Rosen G, Murphy ML, Huvos AG, et al: Chemotherapy, *en bloc* resection, and prosthetic bone replacement in the treatment of osteogenic sarcoma. Cancer 37:1–11, 1976
11. Watts HG: Introduction to resection of musculoskeletal sarcomas. Clin Orthop 153:31–38, 1980
12. Pritchard DJ, Dahlin DC, Dauphine RT, et al: Ewing's sarcoma: a clinicopathological and statistical analysis of patients surviving five years or longer. J Bone Joint Surg [Am] 57:10–16, 1975
13. Enneking WF, Kagan A: "Skip" metastases in osteosarcoma. Cancer 36:2192–2205, 1975

CHAPTER 5

PRINCIPLES OF CHEMOTHERAPY

John H. Edmonson, M.D.
Gerald S. Gilchrist, M.D.

General Principles

The purpose of cytotoxic drug treatment in bone tumors, as in other cancers, is the selective destruction of cancer cells. Unfortunately, most current cancer chemotherapy is not specifically tumoricidal but rather is cytocidal for cells of various origins which are engaged in mitotic replication. Only a very few cytotoxic drugs are significantly cytocidal for resting noncycling cells, although metabolic poisoning and temporary impairment of cell functions are not uncommon after exposure of even totally nondividing cells, such as neurons and skeletal muscle cells, to certain cytotoxic drugs. Antitumor drugs are active in destroying normal human cells from tissues that continuously maintain significant pools of actively proliferating cells; thus bone marrow, hair follicles, skin and mucous membranes, enteric epithelium, and germinal epithelium may share with the cancer cell targets many of the cytotoxic effects of cancer chemotherapy. For this reason, the selection of drugs for clinical cancer chemotherapy must emphasize the therapeutic index rather than simply the destruction of cancer cells alone.

Obviously, to be effective, antitumor drugs must be administered in a manner that permits the optimal exposure of the cancer cells to the drug or drugs. The physicochemical properties of each drug influence its distribution within the various body compartments that harbor cancer cells. These properties also may determine the most effective route and rate of administration, for example, by rapid intravenous injection or prolonged infusion or by oral administration. If special pharmacologic "sanctuaries" are involved by the cancer, special methods may be required in order to expose the cancer cells to cytocidal drug concentrations, for example, intrathecal treatment for disease of the central nervous system. Efforts to produce optimal exposure of cancer cells to antitumor drugs will necessarily also consider the distribution and size of the tumor burden present and all available information concerning the expected level of sensitivity of the given cancer cell type to cytotoxic drugs.

In an attempt to enhance the tumoricidal effects, different drugs known to be individually active against a particular type of tumor have been combined to produce a combination of biochemical lesions. To maintain optimal cell kill, efforts are made to use as near full doses of each drug as possible: thus agents that have different dose-limiting toxic actions are most often combined.

Following the work of Skipper and his colleagues (1), the log kill principle for sensitive cells has been widely accepted as the basis for tumor reduction by cytotoxic agents. According to this principle, each dose of the cytotoxic regimen destroys a certain percentage of the sensitive cancer cells, and if all cells remain sensitive to the treatment, cure can be predicted for regimens that are able to kill cancer cells more rapidly than the surviving cells are able to proliferate. These investigators and others have demonstrated that small tumor foci are much more likely to be destroyed by chemotherapy than are large masses. Unfortunately, cancer cells resistant to chemotherapy are extremely common, and resistant clones will often emerge during the treatment of tumors that initially seemed to be quite sensitive to drug treatment. Goldie et al (2) have studied this process extensively and have developed a rational approach to combat the emergence of mutationally engendered chemotherapy-resistant cells. These investigators have provided mathematic support for the alternating use of non-cross-reacting effective regimens when the patient is unable to tolerate all of these different active agents together. The treatment of micrometastases (adjuvant chemotherapy) requires the same optimal cytotoxic regimens as those required in advanced cancers; however, the treatment may not need to be prolonged.

The specific choice of drugs (and doses) for the treatment of cancer in an individual case also may be affected by factors that modify the metabolism of specific chemotherapeutic agents. For example, young children tolerate vincristine and methotrexate quite well, whereas patients with hepatic, cardiac, or renal dysfunction may tolerate certain agents poorly if given in usual doses. Organ dysfunction may affect the metabolism of individual cytotoxic drugs, and the concomitant administration of multiple cytotoxic agents or their use with other drugs may also alter drug action.

Specific Examples

Certain rapidly proliferating malignant tumors such as Ewing's sarcoma are often exquisitely sensitive to cytotoxic drugs, with some patients who have this disease being cured despite the presence of widespread metastasis. Chondrosarcomas, at the other extreme, are most often totally drug-resistant, although mesenchymal chondrosarcoma may be quite sensitive to drug treatment. Osteosarcomas, malignant fibrous histiocytomas, and fibrosarcomas of bone tend to have drug-sensitive characteristics that lie somewhere within a broad spectrum separating the two extremes among malignant bone tumors. Other less common types of bone tumors—for example, metastasizing "benign giant cell tumors"—may on occasion regress under the influence of cytotoxic drugs; however, little is known of the usefulness of cancer chemotherapy in most of the rare malignant bone tumors. Generally, low-grade sarcomas and benign tumors of bone are not treated with cytotox drugs; however, eosinophilic granuloma, a neoplasia-like disease, may require systemic chemotherapy in its more disseminated forms.

Chemotherapy has been utilized in the treatment of bone tumors after the recognition of overt metastasis; however, during the past decade, patients with apparently localized Ewing's sarcoma and osteosarcoma have had cytotoxic drugs introduced soon after primary surgery or radiation and at times even prior to other treatment (see illustrative case 1). Definite survival benefits seem to result from this adjuvant chemotherapy in patients with Ewing's sarcoma and perhaps in those with osteosarcoma; however, no randomized controlled clinical trial has yet proved this benefit in patients with osteosarcoma.

As might be said concerning most types of cancer treatment in the early 1980's, the chemotherapy of bone tumors is still largely investigational, with various drug regimens under study. Most of these treatment regimens include a combination of agents, and most currently include doxorubicin. Other single agents that have proved to be useful in combination treatment regimens are alkylating agents such as cyclophosphamide, melphalan, cisplatin, and mitomycin, the antimetabolite methotrexate, as well as vincristine, dacarbazine, and dactinomycin. Bleomycin has also been included in some antineoplastic regimens for bone sarcomas; however, its role remains uncertain at the present time.

The current role of cytotoxic drugs in the management of bone sarcomas is complementary to that of surgery or radiation therapy (or both), with greater emphasis on these latter two modalities for the control of the primary tumor. Chemotherapy serves best in the destruction of small metastatic lesions, but in some situations it may also initiate the control of locally extensive disease and its systemic symptoms. Patients who are anorectic, febrile, and ill as a result of rapidly proliferating sarcomas may be improved dramatically by systemic chemotherapy, thus facilitating the treatment of their primary tumors, perhaps allowing more effective use of surgical and radiation treatments of these lesions (see illustrative case 2).

The apparent clonal heterogeneity of bone sarcomas may lead to variable efficacy of cytotoxic drug treatments in different lesions within the same patient, with some metastatic lesions regressing at a time when others are stable and still others are growing. The use of two or more non-cross-reacting drug regimens may overcome some of this clonal variation in drug sensitivity. The clinical emergence of a previously unrecognized resistant cell line may produce focally progressive disease in some more rapidly growing tumors, for example, Ewing's sarcoma, after only 2 or 3 months of otherwise successful treatment (see illustrative case 2). Thus, careful follow-up examination with appropriate shifts in therapy when indicated is an essential feature of the treatment of bone sarcoma, and the careful integration of surgical and radiation therapies with chemotherapy is a critical requirement for success.

Illustrative Cases

Case 1. A 16-year-old schoolgirl experienced pain in her right knee 3 weeks before coming to the Mayo Clinic. Roentgenograms taken in her home community were suspicious for osteosarcoma of the distal femur. Surgical biopsy of the distal right femur revealed a grade 3 chondroblastic osteosarcoma. A computed tomographic scan of the chest was normal, and bone scan revealed uptake only at the right femoral tumor site. Femoral roentgenograms indicated the existence of some extension medially through the cortex of the femur.

Chemotherapy was given preoperatively in the hope of utilizing limb-sparing surgery (Fig. 5-1 *A*). A combination of bleomycin, cyclophosphamide, doxorubicin, and cisplatin was given in four monthly courses before surgery, with relief of symptoms, decline of serum alkaline phosphatase levels, and increasing tumor mineralization (Fig. 5-1 *B*). A fibermetal implant was inserted with a knee arthrodesis after wide excision of the right distal femur. The patient was able to return to school and has received no further chemotherapy.

Case 2. A 24-year-old woman experienced pain in her right hip and groin several weeks before coming to the Mayo Clinic. She also had noted swelling in the right inguinal region and thigh of 1 week's duration. She was anorectic, febrile, and in pain. Surgical biopsy of the inguinal mass revealed Ewing's sarcoma, which on a roentgenogram was found to involve the anterior and posterior right pubic rami and to displace the bladder medially. Metastasis to the right lung, the proximal femur,

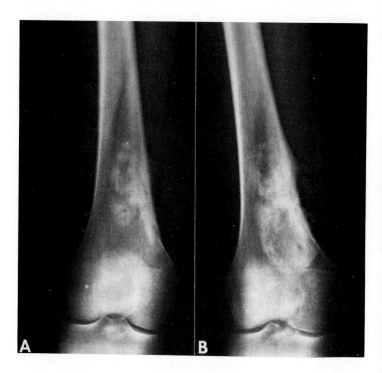

Fig. 5-1.(case 1). Grade 3 chondroblastic osteosarcoma of distal right femur. *A*, Before chemotherapy. *B*, After four courses of chemotherapy.

Bone Tumors

the cervical spinal column, and the skull was identified on a chest roentgenogram and a radionuclide scan of the skeleton.

After one course of combination chemotherapy with mito-mycin, doxorubicin, and cisplatin, the fever resolved, the mass regressed, and her appetite began to improve. When she returned after 1 month, her pulmonary lesions had completely regressed and she had begun walking again. After the second course of this chemotherapy, roentgenograms revealed some bony healing of the osteolytic disease, and the pelvic mass was no longer palpable. Unfortunately, a previously uninvolved site, the anterior iliac spine on the right, had become painful and tender, and on a surgical biopsy specimen, partially necrotic Ewing's sarcoma was identified. At this point, she was given radiation therapy to the right anterior pelvis and chemotherapy was continued. Four months after diagnosis, the drug therapy was changed to monthly courses alternating between vincristine, dactinomycin, cyclophosphamide and vincristine, doxorubicin, dacarbazine; however, the disease progressed despite this effort.

References

1. Skipper HE, Schabel FM Jr, Wilcox WS: Experimental evaluation of potential anticancer agents. XIII. On the criteria and kinetics associated with "curability" of experimental leukemia. Cancer Chemother Rep 35:1–111, 1964
2. Goldie JH, Coldman AJ, Gudauskas GA: Rationale for the use of alternating non-cross-resistant chemotherapy. Cancer Treat Rep 66:439–449, 1982

CHAPTER 6

PRINCIPLES OF RADIOTHERAPY

Alvaro Martinez, M.D.

Since the discovery of x-rays by Röntgen and radium by Madame Curie, ionizing radiation, as a therapeutic modality, has been applied mostly in the treatment of "malignant tumors." Kilovoltage equipment (orthovoltage units), originally used to treat patients who had cancer, has virtually disappeared from modern radiotherapy facilities and is no longer employed, except for the treatment of patients with skin cancers. During the last 20 years, the equipment and paraphernalia utilized to irradiate patients have undergone tremendous technological changes. Much knowledge has been accumulated with regard to the biologic effects of megavoltage irradiation on tumors and normal tissues. The use of computers has increased not only the speed of dose calculations but also their accuracy. The routine use of simulators, immobilization devices, and beam modifiers, such as wedge filters and compensators, has improved the quality and reproducibility of daily treatments. Radiotherapy techniques and dose delivery schedules have had particular emphasis, with many publications directed toward maximizing the control of the tumor and minimizing the toxicity to the surrounding normal tissue (1-32).

Only a few concepts on the physical aspects of radiation will be reviewed here. The chapter written by Evans and Donaldson, "Principles of Radiation Biology and Radiation Therapy," in *Cancer in the Young* (33), provides a more complete review.

Basic Concepts

Depending on the electromagnetic charge and penetration, ionizing radiation is classified into four types: (1) alpha rays, which can penetrate only a few centimeters of air or a few sheets of paper, (2) beta particles, which are similar to electrons and which can penetrate up to 4 mm of tissue, (3) gamma rays, which are similar to x-rays but which are given off by radioactive materials that are trying to attain stability, and (4) x-rays, which are artificially produced by bombarding a target with high-speed electrons in a vacuum. In external-beam therapy, we utilize only the "x-rays" produced by high-energy machines (megavoltage). Some substances are radioactive, for example, polonium and radium, and these are called "natural" isotopes. In clinical medicine, the radioisotopes used are generally man-produced in nuclear reactors or cyclotrons. They decay by the production of beta particles or gamma rays.

Units

The National Bureau of Standards, in Handbook 87, thoroughly discusses the measurements of ionizing radiation (34). "Exposure" is the amount of radiation to which a particular object has been exposed, without reference to the nature of the particular material in which the radiation is absorbed (35). The roentgen (R) is the unit of exposure and is the amount of x-ray or gamma radiation that produces an ionization in air of one electrostatic unit of charge (of either sign) per cubic centimeter of air at standard temperature and pressure (22). "Absorbed dose" is the dose of radiation that is delivered to a particular material at the point of interest. The rad is the unit of absorbed dose and is equal to the amount of ionizing radiation that delivers 100 ergs/g of absorber. The unit of radioactivity is the curie (Ci), which is equal to 3.7×10^{10} disintegrations per second. The curie is used to describe the activity of any radioisotope, and it is approximately the equivalent of the number of disintegrations per second undergone by 1 g of radium (23).

Dose

The dose delivered to a patient is expressed in several ways. The maximal or "given" dose is the dose at the point of maximal electronic equilibrium which occurs below the skin. The depth of this point is dependent on beam energy, that is, 1.5 cm for a 6-million electron volt (meV) linear accelerator and 4 cm for a 22-meV accelerator (23,35). The tumor dose, in general, is the dose delivered to a point within or around the tumor (31). The integral dose is the total absorbed dose integrated over the entire body, that is, the total energy absorbed by the entire volume of the patient during irradiation (27). Isodose curves are two-dimensional representations of the distribution of radiation in a particular plane. They can be obtained by direct measurements (irradiating water phantoms) or by mathematical calculations (13,19,23,35).

Equipment

Specific characteristics of the different therapy machines can be obtained from textbooks (14,23,35). Orthovoltage x-ray machines have no use in clinical radiotherapy, with the exception of their use in treating skin cancer. Units that use cobalt-60 are an improvement over orthovoltage units but have significant limitations and limited application. Linear accelerators are high-energy electron accelerators that can be utilized as either electron or x-ray sources. Because this megavoltage equipment has a high output, the real treatment time is short. The beam is very homogeneous, and the penumbra region is very small when compared with that of the cobalt-60 units. The betatron, which also is a megavoltage machine, accelerates the electrons in a circular tube, which is the main difference from the linear fashion of the previously described machines. Both linear accelerators and betatrons can be utilized as electron sources. The main difference and advantage of electrons when compared with x-rays (photons) is that the electrons have a finite range in tissue penetration which is dependent on their energies. Currently, these two types of machines, particularly the linear accelerator, are the machines most used in radiotherapy (Table 6-1).

Interstitial Therapy

Brachytherapy is the treatment of malignant tumors utilizing radioactive sources placed at short distances. Often, it is advantageous to treat a tumor with a radiation source that is directly implanted into the tumor. One of the main advantages of interstitial therapy is its ability to deliver localized high doses of radiation with a sharp falloff of the radiation dose. This falloff permits sparing of normal structures, either the growing tissues of a child or the normally functioning organs of an adult, from the deleterious effect of high-external-beam doses (36–38).

Tolerance of Different Tissues

Our present knowledge of the radiation tolerance of different tissues has been accumulated empirically from clinical studies. Rubin and Casarett (20) have published extensively on the tolerance of various organs for fractionated irradiation (Fig. 6-1).

Lesions Discussed

Various benign and malignant primary bone neoplasms, as well as metastatic spread of tumors to bone, are seen by the

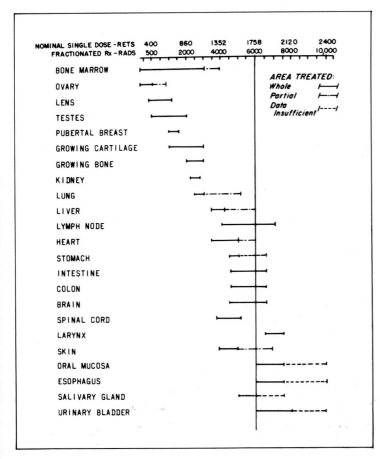

Fig. 6-1. Graphic representation of tolerance doses of fractionated irradiation for various organs. (From Perez CA: Basic concepts and clinical implications of irradiation therapy. *In* Clinical Pediatric Oncology. Edited by WW Sutow, TJ Vietti, DJ Fernbach. St. Louis, CV Mosby Company, 1973, pp 28–70. By permission.)

radiation oncologist. The role of irradiation in the treatment of the more frequently encountered clinical problems will be discussed.

Histiocytosis X. This disease is primarily one of childhood and is expressed in many forms and degrees of virulence. A single lytic bony lesion that clears with very little treatment may be contrasted with a disorder that is unresponsive to therapy, involving multiple organ systems and leading to the death of the patient. Histiocytosis X can be confused clinically and radiologically with either a malignant bone tumor or an infection. Several forms of this disease process can be radiated. In a young child with Hand-Schüller-Christian disease, radiation treatment of a mass in the long bone, vertebra, or soft tissue may be necessary. The mastoid region is often bilaterally involved, and routine radiation treatment can be given on both sides. In the patient with diabetes insipidus, irradiation of the hypothalamic and pituitary regions may reverse the process, providing the treatment is initiated soon after the symptoms appear. In patients with mandibular or maxillary involvement, early treatment may prevent major dental problems, including loss of teeth. Solitary eosinophilic granuloma of bone or soft tissues (or both) is usually seen in children 4 years old or older; however, it also can be seen in adults. The adult form probably is quite different in its clinical behavior and response to radiotherapy when compared with the pediatric form. The use of radiation therapy is recommended after surgery when the disease recurs in surgically inaccessible sites or in a weight-bearing area, where the risk of fracture is high.

The recommended dose levels of irradiation are between 450 and 1,200 rads in the pediatric age group and significantly higher for the adult, that is, 3,000 rads. In Hand-Schüller-Christian disease, doses of 600 rads are enough for control, and Smith et al. (39) reported no local failures after the use of 900 rads. In eosinophilic granuloma, the radiation dose seems to be both age- and site-dependent. In young children with partially resected disease in a flat bone, 450 to 600 rads should be sufficient for local control. However, in the older child with a lesion in a surgically inaccessible weight-bearing region such as the spinal column, higher doses of between 1,000 and 1,200 rads may be necessary to achieve permanent local control. In general, a dose of 600 rads given in three fractions is sufficient for control (40–43). The use of megavoltage equipment is recommended. The radiation fields should be small and tailored to the amount of involvement, with little margin around.

Aneurysmal Bone Cysts. Biesecker et al (44) described the pathogenesis of this lesion as a primary lesion of bone initiating an osseous arteriovenous fistula and thereby creating, via its hemodynamic forces, a secondary reactive bone lesion called an "aneurysmal bone cyst." Radiographically, this lesion presents characteristics similar to those seen in the giant cell tumor, but it affects a younger age group (45). Long bones are the most frequently affected sites, followed in frequency by pelvis and spinal column. Although usually used for the treatment of recurrent disease, radiation therapy also has been given as primary treatment, with local control rates reported in retrospective analyses by both Biesecker et al (44) and Nobler et al (45) as being comparable to those with curettagel with or without bone grafting. Radiation doses of between 2,000 and 3,000 rads given over a period of 20 to 30 days are recommended (44,45). Megavoltage equipment with shaped blocks and multiple-field arrangement should be utilized. My preference is for surgical treatment, reserving radiation for unresectable lesions or first recurrence (or both).

Giant Cell Tumors. Since the recognition of giant cell tumor in 1818, controversy and strong opinions surround its natural history, pathology, and appropriate therapy. In contrast to other bone tumors, giant cell tumors affect females more frequently than males. The peak incidence is around the third decade of life. Histopathologically, most giant cell tumors are benign, and the percentage of malignant variants ranges from 8.7% in the Mayo Clinic series (46) to 30% in the Memorial Hospital series (47). Of clinical relevance are the reports of "metastasizing" benign giant cell tumors of bone (48,49). Curettage with or without bone grafting and complete excision of the primary lesion are the most common surgical procedures utilized in the treatment of these lesions. However, local recurrences rates of 42 to 75% have been consistently reported in large series (46,47,50). A wide range of local failures after irradiation also has been noted (46,47,50,51). The interpretation of reports on radiation therapy has been compromised by the early practice of delivering relatively small doses per fraction over periods of months to years and by the utilization of orthovoltage equipment, with the well-established drawbacks of significant increase in absorbed dose by normal bone (up to three times the stated exposure dose), the inability to treat deep-seated lesions, and the dose-limiting factor imposed by high skin dose.

The malignant transformation of a benign giant cell tumor has been observed in patients treated either by surgery alone or by surgery and irradiation. The studies that were directed to answer the question "Was irradiation the cause of the malignant transformation of a benign giant cell tumor?" have all been retrospective, full of many inaccuracies and lacking appropriate statistical analysis (46,47). No attention has been placed on describing the type of radiation, energy utilized, time-dose factors, or any of the radiation parameters that should be considered when one is trying to postulate a cause-effect relationship. The above historical reports of malignancy developing after irradiation probably represent an "amalgam" of (1) giant cell lesions that were initially malignant but were interpreted pathologically as benign, (2) initially malignant lesions such as fibrosarcomas incorrectly interpreted as benign giant cell tumors, (3) initially benign giant cell tumors that eventually will become malignant, where the radiation was only coincidental, such as when the interval between the irradiation and the malignant transformation was short (in humans, an average of $4^1/_2$ to 5 years is required for a radiation-induced tumor to develop), and (4) the true radiation-induced tumors. The irradiation technique employed at that time to treat this historical group utilizing orthovoltage equipment with preferential bone absorption (3:1 over soft tissue) and the practice of administering small doses of irradiation over a long period may have maximized the "neoplastic potential" of radiation therapy.

Surgery is recommended as the initial management whenever possible, and radiation is reserved (1) for surgically inaccessible or poorly accessible sites such as spinal column or sacrum, (2) when functional disability would be great after surgery, (3) when complete tumor removal is not possible, and (4) in selected cases after local recurrence. The recommended dose is 4,500 to 5,500 rads given over 5 to $6^1/_2$ weeks. The radiation field should encompass the bone lesion and any soft-tissue extension, with a little margin. Rotational arcs or other multiple-field arrangements (or combinations of these) should be utilized to minimize the adverse effects on normal tissues. Immobilization devices, compensators and wedge filters, routine simulation, and port films with megavoltage units are essential to maximize the results. Cassady (52) and other authors called attention to a paradoxical radiographic increase in apparent tumor extent during radiotherapy or early in the follow-up. When observed over a period of weeks to months, the "extension" almost invariably showed ultimate healing. This phenomenon is also commonly seen in Ewing's sarcoma, skeletal lymphoma, soft-tissue sarcomas, and other invasive lesions.

Tumors of Vascular Origin. The literature on malignant vascular tumors is confusing, partly because of problems with nomenclature and partly because of the rarity of the tumors. In Unni and co-workers' (53) review of more than 4,000 bone tumors from the surgical files of the Mayo Clinic, only 69 bone tumors of vascular origin were found. These included tumors from patients operated on at the Clinic and lesions that were sent for review. Hemangiomas were the most frequently seen tumors, with an almost 2:1 female-to-male ratio. Local pain or swelling (or both) was the most common presenting symptom. The skull and vertebra were by far the most frequent sites involved. Ten of the 13 patients with vertebral hemangiomas presented with signs of cord compression. Radiotherapy was used in 7 of the 13 patients, and 6 of the 7 had good responses to treatment. In the patients with hemangioendotheliomas, the most reliable indicator of prognosis was the grade of anaplasia. The authors concluded that the choice of treatment for bone tumors of vascular origin depends on the location of the tumor. Complete surgical removal should be employed when feasible. Radiation therapy is valuable for tumors that are surgically inaccessible or that have not been removed completely.

The recommended dose for spinal lesions is related to spinal cord tolerance, 4,000 to 4,500 rads in 6 weeks. Megavoltage units should be utilized. The arc-wedge technique, for example, has many technical advantages in the treatment of spinal lesions (54). For lesions in locations other than the spinal column, higher radiation doses of 5,000 to 5,500 rads should be utilized. Multiple-field arrangement using megavoltage units is advised.

Non-Hodgkin's Lymphoma of Bone. This malignant tumor is histologically indistinguishable from malignant lymphoma arising in other regions of the body. By definition, it involves a single site in bone. The lesion tends to spread to lymph nodes and distant sites (including other bones) in an unpredictable fashion. The so-called reticulum cell sarcoma of bone has both radiologic and histologic features that are similar to those of a more commonly seen bone lesion, Ewing's sarcoma. However, the better prognosis in primary skeletal lymphoma is a compelling reason for distinguishing it from the more aggressive Ewing's tumor. The goals of radiation treatment of patients with skeletal lymphoma, as well as the technique, are very similar to those for Ewing's sarcoma, and only the dose levels differ slightly. In the report by Desoretz et al (55) on primary lymphoma of bone, there were no local failures in patients who received doses of more than 5,000 rads, and the cumulative incidence of local recurrence was 15%. In contrast, in the review of the literature by Tefft et al (56), the local control rates for patients with Ewing's sarcoma treated with irradiation doses of between 5,000 and 7,000 rads ranged from 62 to 67%.

Significant differences in the natural history exist between the pediatric and the adult form of non-Hodgkin's lymphoma of bone. In the young, a high incidence of leukemic conversion occurs, as with other non-Hodgkin's lymphomas of childhood. In their series of 179 patients at the Mayo Clinic, Boston et al (57) reported that fewer than 15% of the patients were less than 20 years of age (whereas 70% of the patients with Ewing's sarcoma were that young). The pelvis was most frequently involved, followed in descending order by femur, humerus, ribs, and tibia. In most published series, the lesion is usually monostotic; a small but significant number of patients with multiple bone involvement are seen. Careful planning of the biopsy site is mandatory, so as not to compromise uninvolved tissue, which could be spared from irradiation. A short discussion is worthwhile between the surgeon and the radiation oncologist concerning the site of the incision when the preoperative diagnosis is round cell tumor.

Because the local control rate is very high and because it

usually prevents amputation, radiation therapy is widely recognized as the treatment of choice (52,55,57–60). Skeletal lymphoma arises in the medullary diaphyseal portion of the bone. Consequently, the initial radiation field should include the entire diaphyseal part of the bone. Since it is extremely rare for the epiphysis to be involved, the epiphysis could be spared from radiation. This is particularly true if chemotherapy is to be used concomitantly with radiation, as is the current trend. Unless there is soft-tissue involvement, the soft tissue that surrounds the bone need not be included in the field of radiation. Care should be taken to preserve as much skin and subcutaneous and deep tissue as possible in order to minimize late postradiation sequelae. In patients in whom chemotherapy is not to be used, the entire bone should be irradiated with 3,500 to 4,000 rads during a 5-week period. Megavoltage equipment should be utilized. Often oblique-opposed fields, tightly shaped, provide the most effective dose-sparing arrangement for normal tissues. Immobilization devices and tissue compensators can be used to ensure daily reproducibility and improve dose homogeneity throughout the irradiated volume. After the whole bone has been treated, the radiation field is reduced to the site of known tumor, with 3 cm of margin for an additional 1,000 rads given over 1 week. Finally, a small cone-down, to the area of the tumor only, is used, for an additional 500 rads in three fractions. In children, since the leukemic conversion rate is high, combination chemotherapy should be utilized. In a series of nine children with primary non-Hodgkin's lymphoma of bone (two with multiple bone lesions), Cassady (52) reported a 100% recurrence-free status at follow-up from 6 months to 6 years. There were no local failures. Desoretz et al (55), from the Massachusetts General Hospital, recently reported no local failures when the total tumor dose was more than 5,000 rads. In published series in which chemotherapy was not used after irradiation, the 5- or 10-year survival rates ranged from 35 to 50% (52,58,59).

Ewing's Sarcoma. In Ewing's sarcoma, the uniformly poor results when therapy is directed only at the primary tumor have been well documented, with 5-year survival rates between 5 and 25% (61–64). This poor biologic behavior suggests that most patients with apparently localized disease at diagnosis actually have widespread subclinical metastasis. Clinical trials at various institutions have revealed that Ewing's sarcoma, having metastasized, was sensitive to many chemotherapeutic agents, but eventually the disease recurred and caused death, although survival was prolonged by the use of chemotherapy. At diagnosis, the high probability of widespread subclinical disease and the recognition of adequate chemotherapy responses to metastatic disease led to the use of systemic therapy as an adjuvant to eradicate microfoci of disease. In 1969, Johnson and Humphreys (65) demonstrated the beneficial effects of adjuvant chemotherapy when combined with local radiotherapy. In 1972, Hustu et al (66) reported on 15 patients who had localized Ewing's sarcoma treated with cobalt-60 teletherapy and systemic chemotherapy. All 15 patients experienced complete remission, and 12 of the 15 had survived from the time of diagnosis to the time of the report. Later, Pomeroy and Johnson (67) reported a 5-year survival of 52% for 43 patients treated with a combined modality. More recently, Cassady (68) reported a 5-year actuarial survival of 65% for patients who, when initially seen, had disease limited to the bone and adjacent soft tissues and were treated by local irradiation and intensive multiple chemotherapy.

In most centers, radiotherapy has been employed as the primary treatment for Ewing's sarcoma because it produces equal or greater numbers of survivors than does ablative surgery, with preservation of function. A carefully planned and executed radiation program is necessary for obtaining the highest degree of tumor control while keeping the incidence and severity of complications to a minimum.

Ewing's sarcoma tends to originate in the medullary portion of the diaphyseal region of the bone. Because transmedullary spread throughout the affected bone occurs, the entire bone should he irradiated during most of the treatment course, although this may not be necessary. During the last few years, my approach has been to irradiate the tumor and the adjacent soft-tissue involvement with moderate margins around it. Both epiphyseal centers are spared from the irradiation beam unless the lesion includes the epiphysis. Whenever possible, an attempt is made to exclude the metaphysis from the irradiation beam.

Suit (69) also challenged the concept of transmedullary spread, pointing out that recurrences in bone not involved originally by tumor are extremely rare. Uninvolved skin and soft tissues must be carefully protected, and special consideration should be given to maintain a significant strip of nonirradiated skin and subcutaneous tissues. This strip should be at least 3 or 4 cm in width in order to prevent the late development of lymphedema and constrictive fibrosis of the extremity. If this strip-saving maneuver cannot be obtained, serious consideration should be given to surgery as primary treatment. Since vascular and lymphatic channels are most abundant in the medial portion of both the upper arm and lower leg, these nonirradiated strips should be located medially when the disease extent permits. Immobilization devices are mandatory for both the initial and the subsequent cone-down fields. Routine use should be made of simulation of the volume to be treated, individually made blocks shaped to the specific clinical situation, computerized isodose plots taken at multiple levels, and, when indicated, individually made compensators to correct for surface irregularities and differences in circumference (2). The time has come when opposed rectangular or square fields are no longer acceptable.

Lymph node involvement does not seem to be a clinical problem in patients with peripheral lesions. Information is not available on centrally located lesions. Of interest is the technique used by Hustu et al (66) for tumors arising in the innominate bone—they treat the entire pelvis and administer lower doses to the para-aortic nodes. With tumors of the thoracic cage, the entire hemithorax is irradiated at a lower dose than the primary site. Few investigators advocate the prophylactic irradiation of the neuroaxis. In multiple clinical trials, using primary radiation therapy and systemic chemotherapy without prophylaxis to the central nervous system, investigators failed to demonstrate a substantial primary central-nervous-system relapse (66,70–72). Therefore, prophylaxis of the central nervous system cannot be recommended.

Radiation treatment should begin 10 days after the first chemotherapy cycle has been completed. The initial treatment dose is 3,600 rads in 20 increments of 180 rads given five times a week. This is followed by 2 weeks without therapy. Successive cone-down fields are then introduced at 3,600 rads, with a 3-cm margin in all directions, and at 5,000 rads, with only a 1-cm margin, for a total tumor dose of 5,500 to 5,800 rads utilizing the concept of shrinking-field technique (2). This part of the treatment is also given at 180 rads per fraction five times per week. All radiation fields should be treated daily to provide homogeneity of the daily tumor dose and to minimize the side effects of radiation. No adjustments in daily dose are made on the basis of the patient's age at the initiation of therapy, but smaller total doses are given to children who are less than 6 years of age. Perez et al (73) reported on 271 patients with nonmetastatic Ewing's sarcoma from the intergroup Ewing's sarcoma study. With more than 1-year follow-up, the preliminary analysis showed an overall primary tumor control of 89%. This represents a significant improvement over the rate from studies utilizing radiotherapy alone. In the reports from Jenkin et al (74) and Suit (75), the local control rates were 33 and 38%, respectively, for patients treated during the prechemotherapy era. Hustu et al (66), Pomeroy and Johnson (67), Rosen et al (70), Fernandez et al (71), and Chabora et al (76) all have reported local control rates of about 90% when intensive multiple-agent chemotherapy and high doses of megavoltage irradiation were given. Cassady (68) has described the potential postradiation complications.

Another alternative for local treatment, advocated by Rosen et al (77), is the surgical removal of the involved bone, that is, clavicle, rib, metacarpal, metatarsal, or fibula. If the tumor is completely removed and no residual disease is left, postoperative radiotherapy is not recommended. Chemotherapy alone should be adequate. If a microscopic residual tumor is left, doses of about 5,000 rads given over a period of 6 weeks with the shrinking-field technique (2) and adjuvant chemotherapy should be adequate.

A major obstacle to satisfactory therapeutic results in the

treatment of Ewing's sarcoma remains the development of distant metastasis, which is seen in almost 50% of the patients (73). The search for more effective chemotherapeutic agents must continue.

Osteogenic Sarcoma. During the last decade, major developments in the management of osteogenic sarcoma have occurred. These include (1) better understanding and definition of the histopathologic criteria, (2) improved staging procedures (routine use of bone scans, chest tomography, and computed tomography), (3) new and improved surgical techniques, and (4) the routine use of adjunctive multiple-agent chemotherapy. It must be stressed that surgical treatment of the primary tumor is considered the treatment of choice. The surgical trend, recently, is toward "limb preservation" with the use of prosthesis in selected cases. However, function continues to be suboptimal in many of these patients.

Twenty-five years ago, Sir Stanford Cade (78), in England, challenged the traditional concept of amputation after the diagnosis of osteogenic sarcoma. He believed that, since 80% of the patients treated by amputation suffered metastatic spread by 1 year, a treatment program of preoperative irradiation and "delayed" amputation should be given in an attempt to decrease the number of ablative surgical procedures. Lee and Mackenzie (79) reported on a series of 92 patients treated with this approach who had a minimal follow-up of 5 years. Strict histologic criteria were utilized. The initial evaluation for metastatic disease was limited to chest roentgenography (tomography was not available at that time). Patients were treated with the 2-meV Van de Graaff machine to a tumor dose of between 7,000 and 8,000 rads, at 1,000 rads per week for 7 to 9 weeks. After a waiting period of 4 to 6 months, patients without evidence of metastatic spread underwent amputation. Also, the patients in whom local recurrence developed before this time underwent amputation. Radical surgery was not performed if the tumor location made surgery unsuitable, if a good response with good function was obtained, or if metastasis developed. Of the 92 patients, 70 died of disease and 22 were alive without disease at 5 years; and 7 of the 20 survivors achieved control with irradiation without surgery. In the subgroup of patients with lesions in the femur, 46 patients were treated and 14 (30%) were alive at 5 years. Five of the 14 received radiation alone, with no amputation. However, of the nine patients who underwent amputation only, two had persistence of tumor demonstrated histologically. Function was maintained, although the quality of the function was not recorded. In the patients with metastatic spread who did not undergo amputations, the rate for local control was not available. Lee and Mackenzie (79) stated that the results were equal to or perhaps even a little better than the best surgical figures. The inference was that nothing is lost by the delay in ablating the irradiated tumor. The patient's fate depends on the presence or absence of indiscernible metastasis that exists at initial presentation.

Caceres and Zaharia (80) gave large daily doses of irradiation, 1,000 to 2,000 rads, to a total dose of of 8,000 to 12,000 rads in 10 to 12 days, followed by immediate surgery. Histologic analysis of the surgical specimens demonstrated that all tumors showed severe radiation damage, 85% of the specimens had extensive areas of necrosis, and 28% of the specimens had no evidence of tumor. No improvement in survival was demonstrated. However, adding local treatment to a disease in which local recurrence after amputation is infrequent should not improve survival. By the use of conventional radiation fractionation, the local control rates are less than 25% (81). This limited effectiveness of a conventional radiotherapeutic approach may be due to the presence of a relatively high number of hypoxic tumor cells (82). In addition, there is laboratory evidence that osteogenic sarcoma cells may have an increased capacity to repair sublethal radiation damage (82). These radiobiologic parameters may explain the fact that conventional radiotherapeutic fractionation (180 to 200 rads per fraction given five times per week) has been successful in producing local control in only a few patients.

Recognizing the poor surgical results for patients with osteogenic sarcoma arising in unfavorable sites, Martinez et al (83) began a combined nonsurgical therapeutic approach that involved the intra-arterial infusion of a radiosensitizer combined with large radiation dose per fraction. The arterial blood supply of the tumor was infused with 5′-bromodeoxyuridine (5-BUdR) 24 hours prior to a dose of 600 rads external beam every fifth day, to a total dose of 4,600 rads. BUdR was used because it produces radiosensitization when incorporated into cellular DNA in place of thymidine both in vivo and in vitro. Adjuvant chemotherapy also was given.

Ten patients were entered in the study. All patients completed both the irradiation regimen and chemotherapy for periods ranging from 4 to 9.5 years. Local control was obtained in 8 of the 10 patients. Metastasis developed in 6 of the 10 patients. However, one patient was alive without evidence of disease 6.5 years after the onset of pulmonary metastasis, following lung irradiation and intensive chemotherapy. In three patients, severe postirradiation fibrosis developed, and two of them required amputation. Tumor was not found in the surgical specimens of these two patients. Seven of the 10 patients had good to excellent function and range of motion until death or at last follow-up. Five patients have survived and five have died. All five who died had extensive metastatic disease, but two also had evidence of tumor at the primary site. One of the two had a lesion of the proximal humerus. While receiving chemotherapy, he suffered a systemic relapse, which was shortly followed by disease activity at the primary site. The second patient never had clinical evidence of recurrence, but autopsy showed, in addition to generalized metastasis, involvement of the primary site. It is not clear if this involvement represented seeding from the metastasis or persistent failure to obtain local control (83).

Despite adjuvant chemotherapy, lung metastasis developed in nearly 40% of the patients. The trials on adjuvant lung irradiation have not shown decisively any advantage in preventing lung metastasis (84,85). Caldwell (86) reported four patients with osteogenic sarcoma and no evidence of metastatic disease in the lungs at diagnosis who received "elective whole-lung irradiation." Three of the four patients were alive without evidence of disease 2 to 4 years after radiotherapy. In the Mayo Clinic study (85), no advantage in survival was demonstrated in the randomized trial; unfortunately, the low doses of radiation utilized and the small numbers of patients in each group may invalidate the conclusions. Van der Schueren and Breur (84) reported the results from the European Radiotherapy/ Chemotherapy Cooperative Group. A total of 86 patients were entered in that randomized study: 44 patients did not receive irradiation to the lungs and 42 received 2,000 rads in 10 days to both lungs. At 5 years, the disease-free survival was 43% for the patients who received elective lung irradiation and 28% for the patients without any adjuvant therapy. The EORTC, in 1978, started a study directed to answer two questions: Is heavy chemotherapy for about 1 year better than simple lung irradiation? And can the potential gains suggested to be present after both of these treatment policies be combined by adding lung irradiation to the initial induction chemotherapy?

Nearly half of the patients with osteogenic sarcoma will develop metastatic disease. In addition, a few patients will present initially with metastatic spread. When metastasis develops, surgery, irradiation, and chemotherapy alone or in combination have been utilized. Beattie (87) and Telander (88) have reported on the management of pulmonary metastases from osteogenic sarcoma by surgical resection. Rosen et al (89) reported on 16 patients with metastatic osteogenic sarcoma lesions who were treated with intensive chemotherapy and irradiation. Thirteen of the 16 patients had responses. Six of the seven patients treated for bone metastasis had excellent relief of pain; in two of these patients, subsequent biopsy showed no tumor. Two of four patients with pulmonary metastasis showed regression of lesions, but in two patients pulmonary fibrosis developed. Radiation to the primary site in the three patients with metastasis resulted in complete response, although one patient has had a local recurrence since that report was published. Two patients received irradiation for spinal cord compression, and each had a complete response (89).

Currently, radiation therapy has a limited but definite role in the treatment of primary inoperable (83) and metastatic (89) osteogenic sarcoma. If the report of the EORTC shows that a combination of multiple-agent chemotherapy and irradiation is

Table 6-1. Characteristics of Radiation Therapy Equipment

	Orthovoltage	^{60}Co	Linear accelerator
Basic components	x-ray tube	Radioactive source	Electron gun, klystron wave guide
Energy	200–400 kVp	1–2 meV	Variable 4–35 meV
Radiation produced	x-rays (photons)	Gamma rays	Photons, electrons
Size of source or target	5–7 mm	1.5–2.5 cm	1–2 mm
Penumbra	Very large	Large	Minimal
Dose rates (rads/min)	At 80 cm, 50–75 (depending on filter)	50–150 (depending on strength of source)	300 to 1,000
Depth of maximal ionization	Skin	0.5 cm below skin	Variable with energy (1 to 5 cm below skin)
Clinical use	Superficial lesions	Intermediate lesions, moderate doses (4,500–5,500 rads)	Deep-seated lesions, high doses (6,000–7,000 rads); electrons used for lesions at known depths

advantageous, the role of radiotherapy in this disease may be broader than is presently considered.

Multiple Myeloma and Solitary Plasmacytoma. During the last decade, little improvement in survival has been realized for patients with multiple myeloma. Although the initial response rate to chemotherapy is high, the patient soon becomes resistant to the drugs and 50% die within 2 years of diagnosis. In this setting, radiotherapy has only a palliative role to (1) prevent fractures when more than 50% of the bone cortex is destroyed by tumor. (2) relieve pain, and (3) promote healing when a pathologic fracture has been surgically treated. Doses of less than 4,000 rads in 4 weeks are recommended, utilizing megavoltage units. Recently, clinical trials investigated the role of whole-body irradiation as a systemic treatment. No data are available at the present time. Whole-body irradiation in single doses of 400 to 800 rads has been utilized by several investigators to control generalized bone pain, and the response obtained by most patients has been good.

In solitary plasmacytoma of either bone or extramedullary origin, radiation therapy is the treatment of choice. The reports from Meyer and Schulz (90), Mendenhall et al (91), and Corwin and Lindberg (92) corroborate this. Few local failures were seen in patients who received more than 5,000 rads. It has been my experience that, in patients with extramedullary plasmacytoma without bone destruction, doses of between 5,000 and 5,500 rads are sufficient for local control. In patients who have significant bone destruction or plasmacytoma of bone, doses of more than 6,000 rads in 7 weeks are necessary for permanent control. The use of multiple-field megavoltage irradiation is strongly recommended. Corwin and Lindberg (92) demonstrated better survival for patients with extramedullary plasmacytoma than for patients with solitary plasmacytoma of bone and postulated that the two entities are different. Controversy exists regarding the natural history of these disease processes. Most investigators believe that these two are "clinical forms" of the spectrum of multiple myeloma and that, with time, the solitary lesions will become generalized.

References

1. Bunting JS: A head and neck immobilisation unit for use with mega-voltage or teletherapy units. Br J Radiol 39:151–152, 1966
2. Martinez A, Donaldson SS, Bagshaw MA: Special set-up and treatment techniques for the radiotherapy of pediatric malignancies. Int J Radiat Oncol Biol Phys 2:1007–1016, 1977
3. Cameron JR, Suntheralingam N, Kenny GN: Thermoluminescence dosimetry. Madison, University of Wisconsin Press, 1968
4. Carlsson C: Determination of integral absorbed dose from exposure measurements. Acta Radiol [Ther] (Stockh) 1:433–458, 1963
5. Cox JR Jr, Gallagher TL, Holmes WF, et al: Programmed console: an aid to radiation treatment planning. In Proceedings of the 8th IBM Medical Symposium. White Plains, New York, IBM, Technical Publications Department, 1967, pp 179–188
6. Laughlin JS: Realistic treatment planning. Cancer 22:716–729, 1968
7. Mallion WE, White DR: Immobilisation of the head in radiotherapy. Br J Radiol 41:236, 1968
8. Mansfield CM, Galkin BM, Suntharalingam N, et al: Three-dimensional dose distribution in cobalt-60 teletherapy of the head and neck. Radiology 93:401–404, 1969
9. Hall EJ: The relative biological efficiency of x–rays generated at 220 kVp and gamma radiation from a cobalt 60 therapy unit. Br J Radiol 34:313–317, 1961
10. Kaplan HS: Proceedings of the Eleventh International Congress, Biologic Foundations of Radiotherapy, Rome, 1965
11. Cohen M: The organization of clinical dosimetry. I. The four stages of clinical dosimetry. Acta Radiol [Ther] (Stockh) 4:233–256, 1966
12. Pollard EC: Physical considerations influencing radiation response. In The Biological Basis of Radiation Therapy. Edited by EE Schwartz. Philadelphia, JB Lippincott Company, 1966, pp 1–30
13. Sterling TD, Perry H, Katz L: Automation of radiation treatment planning. IV. Derivation of a mathematical expression for the per cent depth dose surface of Cobalt 60 beams and visualisation of multiple field dose distributions. Br J Radiol 37:544–550, 1964
14. Tubiana M, Lalanne C-M: Treatment by supervoltage machines—telecurie apparatus. In Modern Trends in Radiotherapy. Vol 1. Edited by TJ Deeley, CAP Wood. London, Butterworth & Co. (Publishers), 1967, pp 232–249
15. Worton RG, Holloway AF: Lithium fluoride thermoluminescence dosimetry. Radiology 87:938–943, 1966
16. Dembo AJ, Bush RS, Beale FA, et al: Ovarian carcinoma: Improved survival following abdominopelvic irradiation in patients with a completed pelvic operation. Am J Obstet Gynecol 134:793–800, 1979
17. Ellis F: Fractionation in radiotherapy. In Modern Trends in Radiotherapy. Vol 1. Edited by TJ Deeley, CAP Wood. London, Butterworth & Co. (Publishers), 1967, pp 34–51
18. Ellis F: Dose, time and fractionation: a clinical hypothesis. Clin Radiol 20:1–7, 1969
19. Fletcher GH: Textbook of Radiotherapy. Philadelphia, Lea & Febiger, 1966, p 21
20. Rubin P, Casarett GW: Clinical Radiation Pathology. Philadelphia, WB Saunders Company, 1968

21. Herring DF, Compton DMJ: The degree of precision required in the radiation dose delivered in cancer radiotherapy. Report no. EMI-216 from Enviro-Med. Inc., La Jolla, California, July 10, 1970

22. International Commission on Radiological Units and Measurements (ICRU): Physical aspects of irradiation. Handbook 85, report 10b. Washington DC, United States National Bureau of Standards, 1962

23. Johns HE, Cunningham JR: The Physics of Radiology. Third edition. Springfield, Illinois, Charles C Thomas, Publisher, 1974

24. Johnson RE, Kagan AR, Hafermann MD, et al: Patient tolerance to extended irradiation in Hodgkin's disease. Ann Intern Med 70:1-6, 1969

25. Lingren M: Techniques for tumor localization. Cancer 22:735-744, 1968

26. Page V, Gardner A, Karzmark CJ: Physical and dosimetric aspects of the radiotherapy of malignant lymphomas. I. The mantle technique. Radiology 96:609-618, 1970

27. Page V, Gardner A, Karzmark CJ: Physical and dosimetric aspects of the radiotherapy of malignant lymphomas. II. The inverted-Y technique. Radiology 96:619-626, 1970

28. Powers WE, Palmer LA, Tolmach LJ: Cellular radiosensitivity and tumor curability. Natl Cancer Inst Monogr 24:169-184, 1967

29. Scanlon PW: Initial experience with split-dose periodic radiation therapy. Am J Roentgenol 84:632-644, 1960

30. Sambrook DK: Split-course radiation therapy in malignant tumors. Am J Roentgenol 91:37-45, 1964

31. Sundbom L, Åsard PE: Tumour dose concept. Acta Radiol [Ther] (Stockh) 3:135-142, 1965

32. Von Essen CF: A spatial model of time-dose-area relationships in radiation therapy. Radiology 81:881-883, 1963

33. Evans RG, Donaldson SS: Principles of radiation biology and radiation therapy. *In* Cancer in the Young. Edited by AS Levine. New York, Masson Publishing USA, 1982, pp 257-282

34. International Commission on Radiological Units and Measurements (ICRU): Clinical dosimetry. Handbook 87, report 10d. Washington DC, United States National Bureau of Standards, 1962

35. Young MEJ: Radiological Physics. Second edition. London, HK Lewis & Co, 1967

36. Martinez A, Goffinet DR, Donaldson SS, et al: The use of interstitial therapy in pediatric malignancies. Front Radiat Ther Oncol 12:91-100, 1978

37. Martinez A, Herstein P, Portnuff J: Interstitial therapy of perineal and gynecological malignancies. Int J Radiat Oncol Biol Phys (in press)

38. Martinez A, Goffinet DR, Fee W, et al: 125 Iodine implants and an adjuvant to surgery and external beam radiotherapy in the management of locally advanced head and neck cancer. Cancer (in press)

39. Smith DG, Nesbit ME Jr, D'Angio GJ, et al: Histiocytosis X: role of radiation therapy in management with special reference to dose levels employed. Radiology 106:419-422, 1973

40. McGavran MH, Spady HA: Eosinophilic granuloma of bone: a study of twenty-eight cases. J Bone Joint Surg [Am] 42:979-992, 1960

41. Arcomano JP, Barnett JC, Wunderlich HO: Histiocytosis X. Am J Roentgenol 85:663-679, 1961

42. Jones JC, Lilly GE, Marlette RH: Histiocytosis X. J Oral Surg 28:461-469, 1970

43. Enriquez P, Dahlin DC, Hayles AB, et al: Histiocytosis X: a clinical study. Mayo Clin Proc 42:88-99, 1967

44. Biesecker JL, Marcove RC, Huvos AG, et al: Aneurysmal bone cysts: a clinicopathologic study of 66 cases. Cancer 26:615-625, 1970

45. Nobler MP, Higinbotham NL, Phillips RF: The cure of aneurysmal bone cyst: irradiation superior to surgery in an analysis of 33 cases. Radiology 90:1185-1192, 1968

46. Dahlin DC, Cupps RE, Johnson EW Jr: Giant-cell tumor: a study of 195 cases. Cancer 25:1061-1070, 1970

47. Hutter RVP, Worcester JN Jr, Francis KC, et al: Benign and malignant giant cell tumors of bone: a clinicopathological analysis of the natural history of the disease. Cancer 15:653–690, 1962

48. Gresen AA, Dahlin DC, Peterson LFA, et al: "Benign" giant cell tumor of bone metastasizing to lung: report of a case. Ann Thorac Surg 16:531–535, 1973

49. Kutchemeshgi AD, Wright JR, Humphrey RL: Pulmonary metastases from a well-differentiated giant cell tumor of bone: report of a patient with apparent response to cyclophosphamide therapy. Johns Hopkins Med J 134:237–245, 1974

50. Larsson S-E, Lorentzon R, Boquist L: Giant-cell tumor of bone: a demographic, clinical, and histopathological study of all cases recorded in the Swedish Cancer Registry for the years 1958 through 1968. J Bone Joint Surg [Am] 57:167–173, 1975

51. Friedman M, Pearlman AW: Benign giant-cell tumor of bone: radiation dosage for each type. Radiology 91:1151–1158, 1968

52. Cassady JR: Radiation therapy in less common primary bone tumors. Prog Pediatr Hematol Oncol 2:205–214, 1979

53. Unni KK, Ivins JC, Beabout JW, et al: Hemangioma, hemangiopericytoma, and hemangioendothelioma (angiosarcoma) of bone. Cancer 27:1403–1414, 1971

54. Larsen RD, Svensson GK, Bjärngard BE: The use of wedge filters to improve dose distribution with the partial rotation technique. Radiology 117:441–445, 1975

55. Desoretz DE, Raymond AK, Murphy GF, et al: Primary lymphoma of bone: the relationship of morphologic diversity to clinical behavior. Cancer 50:1009–1014, 1982

56. Tefft M, Chabora BMcC, Rosen G: Radiation in bone sarcomas: a re-evaluation in the era of intensive systemic chemotherapy. Cancer 39:806–816, 1977

57. Boston HC Jr, Dahlin DC, Ivins JC, et al: Malignant lymphoma (so-called reticulum cell sarcoma) of bone. Cancer 34:1131–1137, 1974

58. Wang CC, Fleischli DJ: Primary reticulum cell sarcoma of bone: with emphasis on radiation therapy. Cancer 22:994–998, 1968

59. Newall J, Friedman M: Reticulum-cell sarcoma. Part II: Radiation dosage for each type. Radiology 94:643–647, 1970

60. Newall J, Friedman M: Reticulum-cell sarcoma. Part III: Prognosis. Radiology 97:99–102, 1970

61. Boyer CW Jr, Brickner TJ Jr, Perry RH: Ewing's sarcoma: case against surgery. Cancer 20:1602–1606, 1967

62. Bhansali SK, Desai PB: Ewing's sarcoma: observations on 107 cases. J Bone Joint Surg [Am] 45:541–553, 1963

63. Phillips RF, Higinbotham NL: The curability of Ewing's endothelioma of bone in children. J Pediatr 70:391–397, 1967

64. Pritchard DJ, Dahlin DC, Dauphine RT, et al: Ewing's sarcoma: a clinicopathological and statistical analysis of patients surviving five years or longer. J Bone Joint Surg [Am] 57:10–16, 1975

65. Johnson R, Humphreys SR: Past failures and future possibilities in Ewing's sarcoma: experimental and preliminary clinical results. Cancer 23:161–166, 1969

66. Hustu HO, Pinkel D, Pratt CB: Treatment of clinically localized Ewing's sarcoma with radiotherapy and combination chemotherapy. Cancer 30:1522–1527, 1972

67. Pomeroy TC, Johnson RE: Combined modality therapy of Ewing's sarcoma. Cancer 35:36–47, 1975

68. Cassady JR: Radiation therapy in Ewing's sarcoma. Prog Pediatr Hematol Oncol 2:191–204, 1979

69. Suit HD: Role of therapeutic radiology in cancer of bone. Cancer 35:930–935, 1975

70. Rosen G, Wollner N, Tan C, et al: Disease-free survival in children

with Ewing's sarcoma treated with radiation therapy and adjuvant four-drug sequential chemotherapy. Cancer 33:384–393, 1974

71. Fernandez CH, Lindberg RD, Sutow WW, et al: Localized Ewing's sarcoma—treatment and results. Cancer 34:143–148, 1974

72. Jaffe N, Traggis D, Salian S, et al: Improved outlook for Ewing's sarcoma with combination chemotherapy (vincristine, actinomycin D and cyclophosphamide) and radiation therapy. Cancer 38:1925–1930, 1976

73. Perez CA, Tefft M, Nesbit M, et al: The role of radiation therapy in the management of non-metastatic Ewing's sarcoma of bone: report of the Intergroup Ewing's Sarcoma Study. Int J Radiat Oncol Biol Phys 7:141–149, 1981

74. Jenkin RDT, Rider WD, Sonley MJ: Ewing's sarcoma: a trial of adjuvant total-body irradiation. Radiology 96:151–155, 1970

75. Suit HD: Ewing's sarcoma: treatment by radiation therapy. In Tumors of Bone and Soft Tissues. Chicago, Year Book Medical Publishers, 1965, pp 191–200

76. Chabora BMcC, Rosen G, Cham W, et al: Radiotherapy of Ewing's sarcoma: local control with and without intensive chemotherapy. Radiology 120:667–671, 1976

77. Rosen G, Caparros B, Mosende C, et al: Curability of Ewing's sarcoma and considerations for future therapeutic trials. Cancer 41:888–899, 1978

78. Cade S: Sarcoma of bone. Ann R Coll Surg Engl 9:211–223, 1951

79. Lee ES, Mackenzie DH: Osteosarcoma: a study of the value of pre-operative megavoltage radiotherapy. Br J Surg 51:252–274, 1964

80. Caceres E, Zaharia M: Massive preoperative radiation therapy in the treatment of osteogenic sarcoma. Cancer 30:634–638, 1972

81. Price CHG, Jeffree GM: Metastatic spread of osteosarcoma. Br J Cancer 28:515–524, 1973

82. Van Putten LM: Tumour reoxygenation during fractionated radiotherapy: studies with a transplantable mouse osteosarcoma. Eur J Cancer 4:173–182, 1968

83. Martinez A, Goffinet DR, Donaldson S, et al: Combined high dose irradiation, intra-arterial infusion of radiosensitizer and chemotherapy for primary treatment of osteogenic sarcoma (submitted for publication)

84. Van der Schueren E, Breur K: Role of lung irradiation in the adjuvant treatment of osteosarcoma. Recent Results Cancer Res 80:98–102, 1982

85. Rab GT, Ivins JC, Childs DS Jr, et al: Elective whole lung irradiation in the treatment of osteogenic sarcoma. Cancer 38:939–942, 1976

86. Caldwell WL: Elective whole lung irradiation. Radiology 120:659–666, 1976

87. Beattie EJ Jr, Martini N, Rosen G: The management of pulmonary metastases in children with osteogenic sarcoma with surgical resection combined with chemotherapy. Cancer 35:618–621, 1975

88. Telander RL, Pairolero PC, Pritchard DJ, et al: Resection of pulmonary metastatic osteogenic sarcoma in children. Surgery 84:335–340, 1978

89. Rosen G, Tefft M, Martinez A, et al: Combination chemotherapy and radiation therapy in the treatment of metastatic osteogenic sarcoma. Cancer 35:622–630, 1975

90. Meyer JE, Schulz MD: "Solitary" myeloma of bone: a review of 12 cases. Cancer 34:438–440, 1974

91. Mendenhall CM, Thar TL, Million RR: Solitary plasmacytoma of bone and soft tissue. Int J Oncol Biol Phys 6:1497–1501, 1980

92. Corwin J. Lindberg RD: Solitary plasmacytoma of bone vs. extramedullary plasmacytoma and their relationship to multiple myeloma. Cancer 43:1007–1013, 1979

Chapter 7

ROLE OF THORACOTOMY IN PRIMARY MALIGNANT BONE TUMORS

Peter C. Pairolero, M.D.
Robert L. Telander, M.D.

Survival of patients with primary malignant bone tumors treated by amputation alone has continued to improve during recent years (1–3), and with improvement in survival, there has been increasing enthusiasm for limb-saving radical resections. However, despite successful treatment of the primary tumor, failure still frequently occurs because of the development of distant metastatic lesions, most of which are occult and not clinically evident at the time of operation for the primary lesion. Most malignant bone tumors spread to the lung before other distant metastatic lesions appear. If the lung lesions are allowed to progress, most patients will be dead within 18 months. Thus, for patients with malignant bone tumors to survive further, an effective method of controlling lung metastasis must be found.

Prophylactic whole-lung irradiation has not improved survival (4). In a randomized prospective study of irradiation to roentgenographically negative lung fields, there was no difference in disease-free survival between control patients and patients who underwent irradiation. Several other important advances, however, have been made in the management of these tumors after amputation. Preliminary reports indicating tumor regression after chemotherapy in patients with metastatic disease were encouraging (5,6) and provided the basis for the introduction of adjuvant chemotherapy for patients without overt metastasis (7,8). Another definite advance has been a more aggressive attitude toward resection of pulmonary metastatic lesions. Although resections of such lesions were first successfully reported by Barney and Churchill (9) in 1939, this procedure was initially reserved only for the patient with a solitary metastatic lesion who had a long tumor-free interval between the onset of the primary tumor and the discovery of the lesion (10). Martini et al (11), however, in 1971, demonstrated the value of multiple pulmonary resections, and since that time, numerous patients have benefited from this procedure (11–14).

In most patients, distant metastasis is limited to the lung, and pulmonary resection can be curative in some. In addition, resection of pulmonary metastatic lesions also can be of value in preventing secondary pulmonary complications, such as the postobstructive pneumonitis and hemoptysis that occur after enlargement of the metastatic lesions. If these complications are allowed to progress, early death ensues.

All patients suspected of having a primary malignant bone tumor should undergo thorough pulmonary evaluation before open bone biopsy. Knowledge of the extent of malignancy can influence the management of the primary bone tumor, as unresectable pulmonary metastatic lesions may preclude amputation. In the past, the lungs were evaluated with plain chest roentgenography and whole-lung tomography. Currently, computed tomography (CT) is a much more sensitive and accurate method of detecting pulmonary metastatic lesions (15).

Both posteroanterior and lateral chest roentgenograms as well as CT should be obtained in all patients at initial evaluation.

Any suspicious lesions found on conventional roentgenography should be further evaluated by the use of localized tomograms. Older patients in particular may have been previously exposed to certain fungal diseases, such as histoplasmosis or coccidioidomycosis, which can lead to the development of pulmonary granulomas. Generally, these granulomas have a smooth, well-defined border and frequently have evidence of central calcification on conventional tomography (Fig. 7-1). Except for calcification, metastatic nodules are similar, and differentiation between the two is difficult (Fig. 7-2). Old chest roentgenograms also should be reviewed, if available, to determine if the suspected lesion had been present previously. If the nodule has been present and unchanged for 2 years, it is extremely unlikely that the lesion is malignant, and such nodules can be safely observed (16). Frequently, however, chest roentgenography is interpreted as normal while CT demonstrates multiple small nodules (Fig. 7-3). These multiple small nodules, especially in the younger patient, are worrisome for the presence of metastatic lesions, and thoracotomy is indicated. If initial lung evaluation does not reveal any suspicious pulmonary nodules, a histologic diagnosis of the bone tumor should be made by a carefully planned open bone biopsy.

If preliminary lung evaluations suggest that a new lung nodule is present, the nodule should be biopsied first. If metastatic bone cancer is discovered and if the lung parenchyma can be rendered tumor-free, definitive treatment of the primary bone tumor should be performed at a later date. If unresectable pulmonary cancer

Fig. 7-1. Benign calcified granuloma. *A,* Posteroanterior view of chest demonstrates 2-cm smooth, well-defined solitary pulmonary nodule in right mid lung field. *B,* Tomogram demonstrates central target calcification.

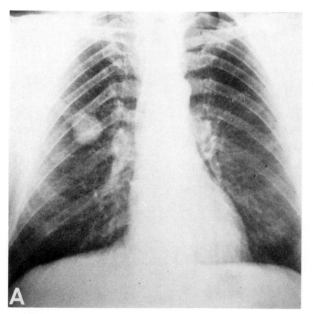

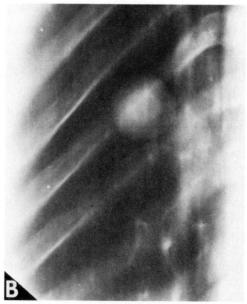

Bone Tumors

is found, consideration should be given to radiation therapy for the primary tumor, which should be followed by chemotherapy.

Generally, a lateral thoracotomy is used to evaluate suspected pulmonary metastasis. However, for bilateral lesions a median sternotomy approach allows a biopsy specimen to be taken simultaneously from each side. The exposure for inspection, palpation, and wedge excision is adequate. Even lobectomy or pneumonectomy can be accomplished through this approach. Previous lateral thoracotomy and large central hilar lesions, however, are relative contraindications to sternotomy.

After assessment of the extent of the disease, wedge excision is generally the preferred method of treatment for the patient with pulmonary metastatic lesions. This procedure allows adequate resection of the nodule without compromising functioning lung parenchyma. Frozen sections are used in all cases to assure that the margins of resection are free of microscopic

Fig. 7-2. Malignant metastatic osteogenic sarcoma. *A,* Posteroanterior view of chest demonstrates 2-cm solitary pulmonary nodule in right mid lung field. *B,* Tomogram demonstrates well-defined nodule. Irregularity in lower medial border is suspicious for malignancy.

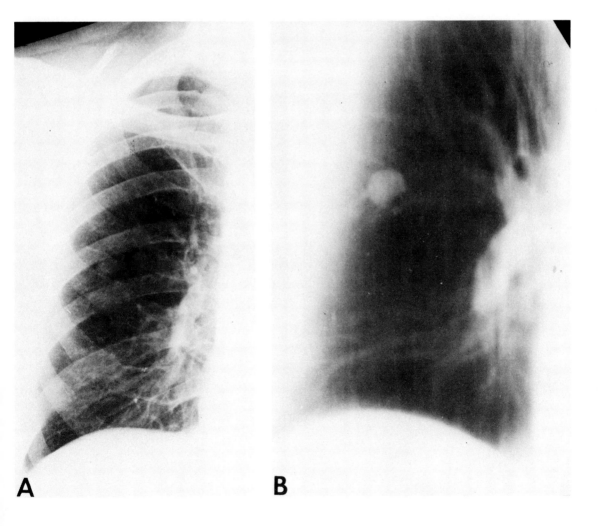

A   **B**

tumor. Sometimes, however, to ensure the total removal of pulmonary metastatic lesions, a segmentectomy, lobectomy, or pneumonectomy may be necessary. Occasionally, extended resections that include portions of the chest wall, diaphragm, or pericardium have been performed, with long-term survival.

After definite amputation, the patient should be reevaluated at 3-month intervals. Subsequent lung evaluation should be similar to the initial evaluation. If new lung nodules are detected, consideration should be given to pulmonary resection. Patients are considered candidates for thoracotomy if the primary bone lesion is under control and there is no evidence of extrapulmonary metastatic disease. The presence of bilateral pulmonary lesions or a short tumor-free interval does not preclude thoracotomy. We do not hesitate to perform multiple-stage thoracotomies if they are indicated.

In our experience, patients with primary bone tumor do benefit from this aggressive approach. The 5-year actuarial survival after thoracotomy in patients with osteogenic sarcoma has been reported as approximately 40% (17,18) (Fig 7-4). Although sur-

Fig. 7-3. Posterolateral (A) and left lateral (B) views of chest of 8-year-old boy. Films interpreted as negative for metastatic pulmonary osteogenic sarcoma. Computed tomography demonstrates two nodules posterolateral (C) and posteromedial (D), which proved to be metastatic sarcoma.

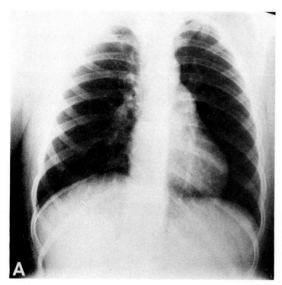

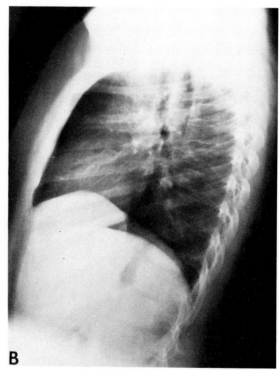

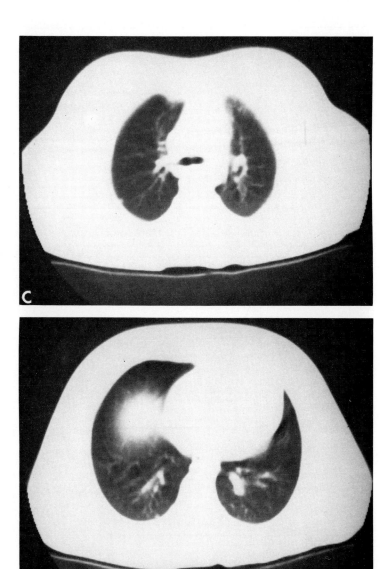

Fig. 7-3

vival was longest for patients with a tumor-free interval of greater than 1 year, 25% of the patients with osteogenic sarcoma who had a tumor-free interval of less than 1 year were still alive an average of 37 months after initial thoracotomy. Approximately 50% of these patients underwent more than one thoracotomy. The number of multiple thoracotomies ranged from 2 to 8, with a mean of 2.9. Of particular importance is that there was no operative mortality and morbidity was limited to one instance of empyema in 111 thoracotomies performed. Postoperatively, patients recovered quickly, with early resumption of normal activity. Similar results were observed in our patients with non-

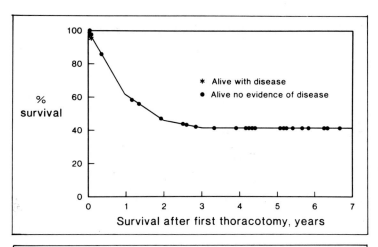

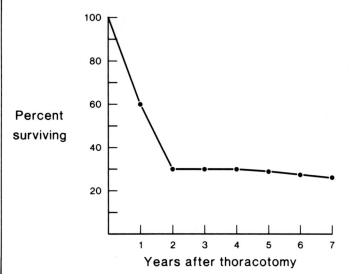

Fig. 7-4. Survival of patients after initial thoracotomy for metastatic osteogenic sarcoma. (From Han M-T, Telander RL, Pairolero PC, et al: Aggressive thoracotomy for pulmonary metastatic osteogenic sarcoma in children and young adults. J Pediatr Surg 16:928-932, 1981. By permission of Grune & Stratton, Inc.)

Fig. 7-5. Survival of patients after initial thoracotomy for nonosteogenic sarcoma.

osteogenic sarcoma. The 5-year actuarial survival after thoracotomy in these patients was 29% (19) (Fig 7-5). On the basis of our experience, we conclude that an aggressive surgical approach to metastatic pulmonary bone tumor is likely to provide a highly effective form of therapy for a large number of patients with advanced disease.

References

1. Sim FH, Ivins JC, Pritchard DJ: Surgical treatment of osteogenic sarcoma at the Mayo Clinic. Cancer Treat Rep 62:205–211, 1978
2. Friedman MA, Carter SK: The therapy of osteogenic sarcoma: current status and thoughts for the future. J Surg Oncol 4:482–510, 1972

3. Taylor WF, Ivins JC, Dahlin DC, et al: Trends and variability in survival from osteosarcoma. Mayo Clin Proc 53:695–700, 1978

4. Rab GT, Ivins JC, Childs DS Jr, et al: Elective whole lung irradiation in the treatment of osteogenic sarcoma. Cancer 38:939–942, 1976

5. Cortes EP, Holland JF, Wang JJ, et al: Doxorubicin in disseminated osteosarcoma. JAMA 221:1132–1138, 1972

6. Djerassi I: High-dose methotrexate (NSC-740) and citrovorum factor (NSC-3590) rescue: background and rationale. Cancer Chemother Rep 6:3–6, 1975

7. Cortes EP, Holland JF, Wang JJ, et al: Amputation and Adriamycin in primary osteosarcoma. N Engl J Med 291: 998–1000, 1974

8. Jaffe N, Frei E III, Traggis D, et al: Adjuvant methotrexate and citrovorum-factor treatment of osteogenic sarcoma. N Engl J Med 291:994–997, 1974

9. Barney JD, Churchill EJ: Adenocarcinoma of the kidney with metastasis to the lung: cured by nephrectomy and lobectomy. J Urol 42:269–276, 1939

10. Clagett OT, Allen TH, Payne WS, et al: The surgical treatment of pulmonary neoplasms: a 10-year experience. J Thorac Cardiovasc Surg 48:391–400, 1964

11. Martini N, Huvos AG, Miké V, et al: Multiple pulmonary resections in the treatment of osteogenic sarcoma. Ann Thorac Surg 12:271–278, 1971

12. Beattie EJ Jr, Martini N, Rosen G: The management of pulmonary metastases in children with osteogenic sarcoma with surgical resection combined with chemotherapy. Cancer 35:618–621, 1975

13. Marcove RC, Martini N, Rosen G: The treatment of pulmonary metastasis in osteogenic sarcoma. Clin Orthop 111:65–70, 1975

14. Rosenberg SA, Flye MW, Conkle D, et al: Treatment of osteogenic sarcoma. II. Aggressive resection of pulmonary metastases. Cancer Treat Rep 63:753–756, 1979

15. Muhm JR, Brown LR, Crowe JK: Use of computed tomography in the detection of pulmonary nodules. Mayo Clin Proc 52:345–348, 1977

16. Pairolero PC, Danielson GK, Johnson J: Benign and malignant neoplasms of the tracheobronchial tree, lungs, and pleura. In Practice of Surgery. Edited by FH Ellis. Hagerstown, Maryland, Harper & Row, Publishers, 1978, pp 1–92

17. Telander RL, Pairolero PC, Pritchard DJ, et al: Resection of pulmonary metastatic osteogenic sarcoma in children. Surgery 84:335–340, 1978

18. Han M-T, Telander RL, Pairolero PC, et al: Aggressive thoracotomy for pulmonary metastatic osteogenic sarcoma in children and young adolescents. J Pediatr Surg 16:928–932, 1981

19. Creagan ET, Fleming TR, Edmonson JH, et al: Pulmonary resection for metastatic nonosteogenic sarcoma. Cancer 44:1908–1912, 1979

CHAPTER 8

LIMB SALVAGE AND RECONSTRUCTIVE TECHNIQUES

Franklin H. Sim, M.D.
William E. Bowman, Jr., M.D.
Edmund Y. S. Chao, Ph.D.

Amputation is the standard surgical treatment for high-grade primary malignant bone tumors (1–7). In the past, limb-saving resection has been successfully used for low-grade malignancies and aggressive benign lesions (8–12). However, these procedures were not used for high-grade malignancies because the local recurrence rate was unacceptably high and adversely affected patient survival (13–15).

In recent years, the survival of patients with primary malignant neoplasms has improved dramatically (16–21). Many observers have attributed this improved prognosis to the use of adjunctive chemotherapy (14,22–27). Others believe that the issue has been clouded by the use of historical controls and that improved survival may be due to a multitude of factors, including earlier diagnosis, more accurate preoperative staging, the recognition of histologic variants, and changes in the biologic behavior of the tumor (17,28–32). Regardless of the reason, the improved prognosis of patients with these high-grade lesions has rekindled interest in a more conservative approach to obtaining local tumor control. At the same time, advances in techniques of oncologic reconstruction offer new methods of managing these large defects created by adequate local resection (33–38).

In this chapter, we address the issues in limb-sparing surgery: Do the functional results justify the risk and morbidity of these procedures, and can they be performed without adversely affecting patient survival?

Historical Perspectives

The earliest reports of limb salvage for bone sarcomas were by Eiselsberg (39) in 1897 and Klapp (40) in 1900. Both authors reported the successful use of bone grafts to repair large defects created by resection of the lesion. After these articles were published, there were numerous case reports, but most of the results were either inconclusive or unsuccessful (19).

Phemister (15) credited Lexer with the first successful results in a series of six patients. Three of the patients were disease-free at 3, 7, and 19 years. Phemister also noted the dismal results in six patients described by Roscher. Five of these patients had early local recurrence and died.

In 1936, Albee (41) reported on 13 patients who underwent limb salvage for bone tumors. Three lesions involved the shoulder girdle, seven were in the distal femur, and three were in the tibia. Four of the 13 patients probably had benign giant cell tumors, but the remainder of the lesions were sarcomas. No local recurrences were noted at a minimum follow-up of $2^1/_2$ years. One patient developed an infection that required amputation, and three patients died from pulmonary metastasis.

In 1940, Phemister (15) reported on seven patients (one with involvement of the mandible) treated by resection and bone grafting. Two patients had local recurrence and died from metastasis. Phemister concluded that, in carefully selected patients, limb salvage was technically possible and was a viable alternative to amputation. In 1945, he reported on an additional two patients who had large bilateral tibial grafts (42).

Although there were sporadic reports of limb salvage in patients with high-grade sarcoma, the procedure was reserved generally for patients with aggressive benign lesions and low-grade malignancies (43–46). As experience in resectional surgery increased, new techniques of oncologic reconstruction were employed. The concept of using allografts in tumor surgery was first introduced by Lexer (47) in 1907. At the same time, Judet (48) performed animal experiments using allografts. This method was popularized by Parrish (49,50) in his report of 21 cases. Mankin et al (51) refined the technique and, in 1976, achieved favorable results in 15 patients followed up for an average of 2 years. In 1980, Hiki and Mankin (52) reported an additional experience with 60 patients. However, with increasing use of adjunctive chemotherapy and its adverse effects on healing, other authors have noted less favorable outcomes (53).

Phemister (15,42) was one of the first to introduce the concept of resection arthrodesis in the United States for the treatment of lesions above the knee. Merle D'Aubigné and Dejouany (54) further refined this technique by using Juvara grafts with the addition of a long Küntscher rod. Their series included nine patients, four of whom had high-grade malignancies. There were two with local recurrence in this group. Wilson and Lance (55) and Enneking and Shirley (56) have reported series using modifications of this technique. In a young active patient, many authors believe that this is the procedure of choice since it provides a stable leg capable of a lifetime of use.

Moore and Bohlman (57) were the first to use a metallic prosthesis after resection of a giant cell tumor of the proximal femur. Their patient functioned well for $1\frac{1}{2}$ years after surgery, until he died from an unrelated illness. In 1954, Kraft and Levinthal (58) reported the use of an acrylic distal femoral prosthesis after resection of a giant cell tumor. With the introduction of total joint arthroplasty, there have been several reports of successful series using these techniques in oncologic surgery (12,59).

Marcove et al (60) reported a series of 19 patients with high-grade malignancies who were given preoperative chemotherapy followed by resection and reconstruction by total femur and total knee replacement. Five of the 19 patients required amputation due to infection (three patients) and local recurrence (2 patients). Follow-up ranged from 3 to 29 months. Sim et al (37) have reported successful results of total joint arthroplasty for tumors in both malignant and metastatic diseases. Gait analysis of these patients who have custom total hips for lesions of the proximal femur shows nearly normal walking patterns (61).

During the past few years, many authors have reported successful results in limb salvage of primary malignant bone tumors. Most series stress the need for the careful selection of patients and longer follow-up before final conclusions can be made.

Preoperative Assessment

When the skeleton is compromised by the presence of a malignant lesion, the treating physician must evaluate the patient thoroughly before deciding if limb salvage is possible (6). The following factors are important: age and functional state of the patient; the nature, cause, and progression of the tumor; the degree of osseous destruction; and the extent of soft-tissue involvement. The various methods that may be used in making these decisions have been outlined in previous chapters.

Technique of Resection

The proper selection of patients is mandatory, and the surgical approach demands careful planning. In metastatic lesions when the aim is palliation and in nonneoplastic conditions, the bone excision is conservative and muscle attachments are preserved. However, in primary bone tumors, the aim is eradication of the disease and the resection must be adequate, according to the well-established principles of oncologic surgery. The biopsy wound must be carefully placed so it can be included at definitive resection. The en bloc resection is done through normal tissues, and the lesion is excised with an envelope of normal muscle.

Resection of a proximal femoral lesion is done with the pa-

Fig. 8-1. Illustration of extent of resection and muscles removed in proximal femoral resection for an osseous lesion.

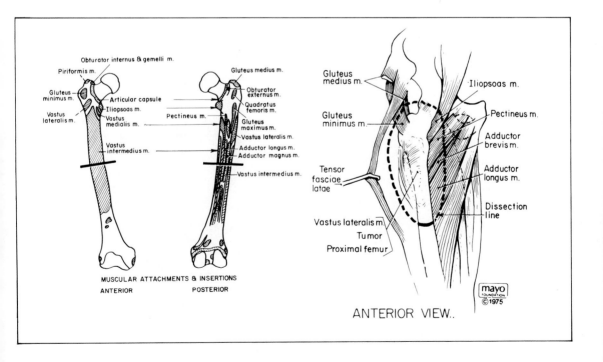

tient in a lateral position in order to obtain wide exposure. The femoral neurovascular structures are isolated anteriorly, and the sciatic nerve is isolated and protected. The length of the proximal femur to be resected depends on the extent of the osseous lesion. The excised muscle mass usually involves the iliopsoas, adductor longus, adductor brevis, gluteus medius, gluteus minimus, and occasionally the gluteus maximus (Fig. 8-1).

Resection of lesions of the proximal tibia or distal femur is done with the patient in the supine position. We prefer a long, medial parapatellar incision, reflecting the patella laterally, but another approach is often dictated by the location of the biopsy incision. Combined medial and lateral incisions may facilitate the resection, and wide skin flaps are necessary for the required exposure. The peroneal nerve, as well as the posterior neurovascular structures, is carefully protected laterally. In tibial lesions, the patellar tendon is detached and reflected upward. The proximal fibula may need to be resected with the specimen. An adequate en bloc resection requires removal of the distal femur or proximal tibia with its surrounding capsule, ligaments, and muscles (Fig. 8-2). Where possible, we do an intra-articular resection because of the improved functional result, but large extracompartmental lesions involving the knee necessitate an extra-articular resection.

Resection of lesions of the pelvis is performed with the pa-

Fig. 8-2. Illustration showing soft-tissue removal in resection of an osseous lesion of the distal femur. Where possible, we prefer to do an intra-articular resection, preserving the patella and rectus femoris to maintain the extension power.

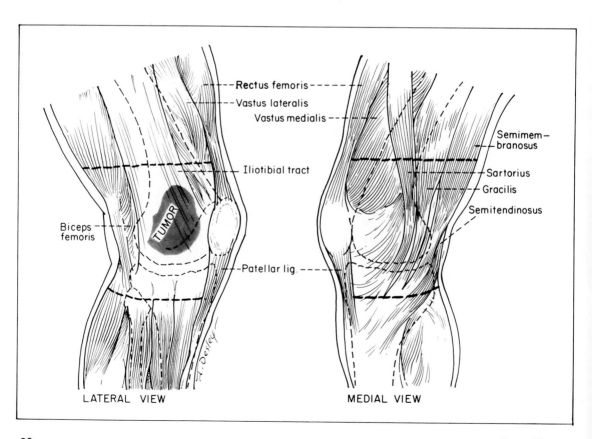

LATERAL VIEW   MEDIAL VIEW

tient positioned for a hemipelvectomy. An extensive exposure is used which provides access to both intra-pelvic and extra-pelvic structures. The incision begins at the posteroinferior iliac spinal column, follows the iliac crest and the inguinal ligament, then turns distally toward the anterolateral aspect of the thigh. If more exposure is needed, the incision may be curved laterally to end posteriorly at the junction of the proximal and middle thirds of the thigh. Furthermore, if the ischiopubic area requires exposure, a supplemental incision may be used along the remaining portion of the inguinal ligament. Large flaps are then developed, and the sciatic nerve and femoral neurovascular structures are identified and protected. The location and size of the lesion dictate the extent of the resection. If the acetabulum is involved, careful preoperative assessment should determine if an extra-articular or intra-articular resection is to be performed. Occasionally when there is a large lesion in the sacroiliac area, hemilaminectomy must be performed to allow adequate resection.

Resection of lesions of the shoulder girdle is achieved with the patient in a semisitting or lateral position (Fig. 8-3). For resection to be successful, preoperative assessment should determine if there is sufficient margin of normal tissue to clear the neurovascular structures. Generally, the Tinkoff-Lindberg incision is used unless a poorly positioned biopsy site requires another incision (40). Large flaps are developed, and, if indicated, the clavicle is resected early to allow exposure of the neurovascular structures. Occasionally, the axillary, radial, or musculocutaneous nerve must be sacrificed to allow for an adequate resection.

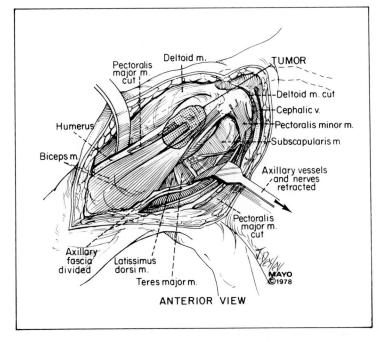

Fig. 8-3. Illustration showing structures involved in resection of osseous lesions in the proximal humerus.

Methods of Reconstruction

Since techniques of oncologic resection have become more refined, we must continue to evaluate and improve our specialized techniques of oncologic reconstruction (14,20,21,27,34). Previously, even if segmental resection of these lesions was possible, the means available to restore the integrity of the bone and joint function in the resected area were inadequate, and little interest was shown in this form of treatment, despite its limb-saving potential. The methods of skeletal reconstruction after radical resection of an osseous lesion vary according to the location of the tumor.

Lesions Involving the Proximal Femur. Previous reconstructive techniques to restore skeletal continuity after radical location resection of osseous hip lesions were plagued by prolonged morbidity and catastrophic complications, such as infections, nonunion, fracture, and disintegration (55,57). In many patients, such as those with a flail extremity, the functional loss was so great that amputation would have been a preferred method of treatment.

Allograft replacement of the proximal femur, unlike that of the knee, has few enthusiasts (49). Bone grafting procedures may obtain an arthrodesis in a shortened extremity. Use of a fibular graft to salvage an immobile joint after resection of a tumor is doomed to failure because of disintegration and collapse (55). However, segmental total hip replacement has been effective in restoring the integrity of the proximal femur and in preserving function of the hip joint (61). These prostheses are presently available in various sizes and lengths, ranging from 80 to 250 mm, so that tumor excision and joint reconstruction can be combined into a single operation (Fig. 8-4).

Lesions Involving the Knee. After resection of the distal femur or proximal tibia, many techniques may be utilized to restore the integrity of the limb (20,33,35,49,50,55,56). When the resection involves removal of only one tibial plateau, the use of the patella to restore the articular surface, combined with autogenous bone graft to restore integrity of the proximal tibia, is an effective means of preserving useful joint function.

Allograft replacement still has many enthusiasts, but it must be considered experimental at this time (14,36,49–52,62) (Fig. 8-5). Although there continues to be a high complication and failure rate, with improvement in the selection and typing, this biologic replacement may gain support. At the present time, work by Mankin and others is encouraging (14,36,49,51,52).

Our preferred method of restoring skeletal continuity after resection of a lesion in the region of the knee, particularly in young persons or in patients with tumors for which the chances of cure are good, is to provide segmental arthrodesis. Although being unable to bend the knee is a functional handicap and

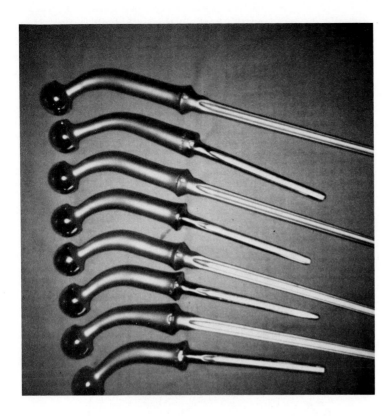

Fig. 8-4. Proximal femoral replacement prostheses. These are now available in lengths ranging from 80 to 250 mm.

inconvenience to the patient, a solid segmental arthrodesis is a definitive procedure that provides a stable, pain-free, weight-bearing extremity. Various methods may be used to achieve this segmental arthrodesis. Enneking et al (63) have used dual fibular grafts combined with an intramedullary rod. We prefer a segmental hemicylindrical sliding graft from the hip's lateral tibia or femur, as described by Merle d'Aubigné and Dejouany (54) (Fig. 8-6).

Another technique that holds much promise is the use of titanium fibermetal implant to restore the integrity of the resected bone. This technique, pioneered by Galante et al (64) has the advantage of not compromising the ipsilateral tibia or the femur and of not compromising the contralateral femur in achieving the segmental replacement (Fig. 8-7).

Utilization of a custom segmental prosthesis with total knee replacement provides an effective means of restoring skeletal continuity in either the distal femur or the proximal tibia while maintaining the function of the knee joint. Because the resection necessitates sacrificing the surrounding soft tissues, joint capsule, ligaments, and dynamic muscular stabilizers, the resulting lack of stability requires a hinged total knee replacement.

Our present segmental replacement hinge arthroplasty consists of a modification of the Walldius total knee replacement. Initially, the size and length of the stem and shaft were individually designed on the basis of the pathologic defect. However, we now have a wide range of sizes available so that the tumor resection and reconstructive procedure can be performed in one operation (Fig. 8-8). We believe that this procedure is

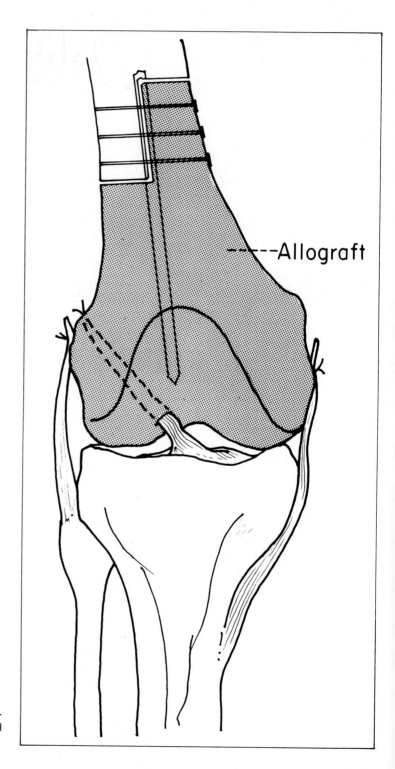

----Allograft

Fig. 8-5. Illustration of technique of allograft replacement to reconstruct distal femur after resection of osseous lesion.

best reserved for older patients, particularly when a cure can be expected by resection of the lesion, such as a benign giant cell tumor. However, the early functional restoration provided by segmental total knee replacement justifies its use as a limb-saving procedure in younger patients who have life-threatening high-grade sarcomas.

Lesions Involving the Shoulder. Various reconstructive methods are available for lesions of the proximal humerus which require resection. The proximal humerus, together with the scapula and clavicle, may be resected according to the method of Lindberg, which leaves the shoulder joint flail (65). Alternatively, one of various bone grafting techniques may be utilized

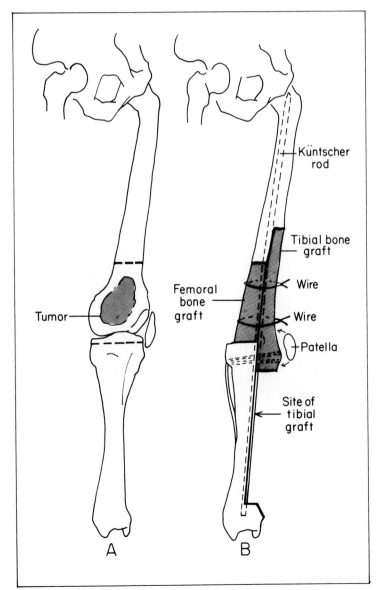

Fig. 8-6. Illustration showing technique of segmental arthrodesis using massive ipsilateral tibial graft and autogenous bone grafts. Fixation is achieved with a long intramedullary rod.

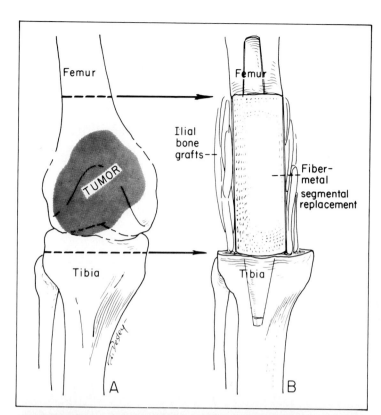

Fig. 8-7. Illustration of technique of achieving segmental arthrodesis utilizing titanium fibermetal composite supplemented by autogenous bone grafts.

Fig. 8-8. Custom distal femoral replacement prostheses. These range from 75 to 200 mm in length.

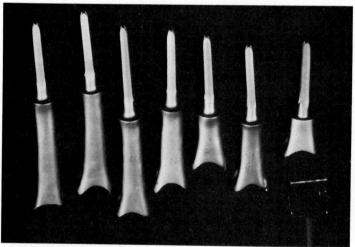

more successfully in this area than in the lower extremity, which is subjected to weight-bearing stresses. Allografts may be useful in this area (Fig. 8-9), but there is insufficient experience to date to warrant utilizing this procedure as a routine method of reconstruction (36,51). The fibula has been used to replace the proximal humerus (55) (Fig. 8-10). In our experience with single fibular replacement, there have been numerous problems due to fracture, nonunion, and disintegration of the graft. Enneking (66) and others have employed dual fibulas in order to avoid

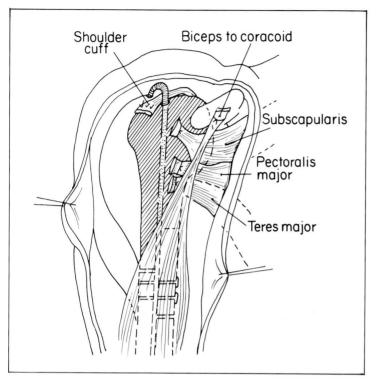

Fig. 8-9. Illustration showing technique of allograft reconstruction of proximal humerus after resection of osseous lesion in the shoulder. This technique has the advantage of biologic fixation of the remaining rotator cuff and soft tissues.

Fig. 8-10. Illustration of techniques utilizing fibular bone graft to reconstruct the proximal humerus after resection of osseous lesions.

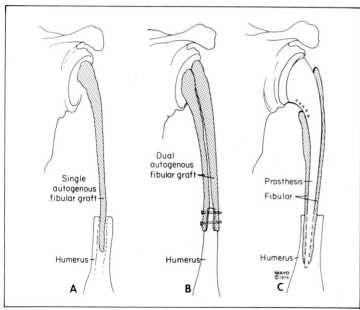

the problem of structural weakness with fracture. With recent advances in microsurgical techniques, a vascularized fibular replacement may be an alternative.

Considerable progress has been made with the use of custom joint implants for the reconstruction of joint function in the shoulder. Previously, we used a ceramic type of humeral replacement. Various sizes of ceramic prostheses are available in stock, and this obviates the previous two-stage procedure. The components include a tapered sleeve, a spacer, and a humoral head (Fig. 8-11). The tapered sleeve is attached extracortically to the conically reamed shaft of the proximal humerus, and this allows for new bone formation and permanent fixation of the implant. After the tapered-sleeve connection has been established, the parts of the prosthesis are joined together with methyl methacrylate (Fig. 8-12). This prosthesis, which was designed by Rosenthal, is no longer being made, but a new design utilizing the fibermetal with the extracortical cone fixation principle is currently being developed.

We are presently using a custom-made Vitallium implant that is essentially an anatomic replacement of the proximal humerus

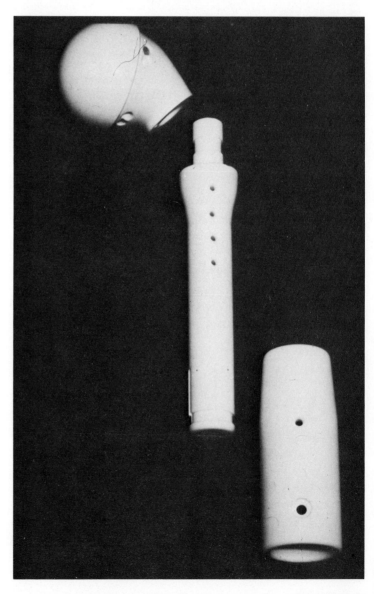

Fig. 8-11. Modular ceramic prosthesis utilized to reconstruct the proximal humerus. Fixation is achieved by fitting the tapered conical sleeve to the conically reamed proximal humerus. Bone ingrowth into the grooves provides permanent fixation.

Bone Tumors

(Fig. 8-13). This implant is also available in various sizes so that a one-stage procedure can be performed.

Lesions of the Pelvis. Various methods of reconstruction have been employed after resection of lesions of the pelvis (67–70). Mankin (71) has used allografts after resection of pelvic lesions, though the final results of these procedures will not be known for several years. There have been various case reports of different prosthetic designs for replacing the hemipelvis (68). We believe that these prostheses may be useful in patients with metastatic disease who have a short life-expectancy. However, in patients in whom the chances of cure are good, these prostheses are doomed to failure because of the biomechanical stresses that will be encountered. With further research into the various alloys and prosthetic designs, this type of prosthesis may become more useful.

The method of reconstruction varies with the relationship of the lesion to the acetabulum and the sacroiliac joint. If a partial resection of the iliosacral area is performed and pelvic continuity is still intact, no reconstruction will be necessary. If the complete iliosacral resection is performed, the remaining portion of the pelvis is hinged on the pubic symphysis and then secured to the sacrum or remaining part of the ilium by wires or screws. Occasionally, autogenous bone grafts also are used. In one instance, we used a vascularized bone graft to reconstruct the defect created by resection of the ilium. After reclosure of the pelvic ring, care must be taken to allow room for the sciatic nerve to exit the pelvis. This usually requires notching the lower portion of the pelvic rim.

In the acetabular region, reconstruction is technically more difficult. If a portion of the acetabular wall is removed, the remaining portion may be reconstructed by the use of autogenous bone grafts. However, if a total acetabular resection is performed, the remaining portion of the femur is usually fused to the ilium (Fig. 8-14) or, in rare instances, to the ischium. If, however, the defect is extremely large and there is not enough remaining bone stock to allow fusion, the femur is left flail. After ischiopubic resection, reconstruction is usually not required unless a portion of the acetabulum is resected.

Diaphyseal Lesions. After resection of the diaphysis of a major bone, a number of reconstructive alternatives exist. Allografts that are secured by plates or an intramedullary rod have been successful in our experience. Dual fibular grafts also may be utilized with various methods of fixation.

During the past several years, we have utilized a titanium fibermetal implant after resection of diaphyseal lesions (Fig. 8-15). This procedure is usually done in two stages. After resection of the lesion, a temporary titanium spacer is placed in the defect. After ascertaining that clear margins of resection are obtained, the prosthetic device is custom-made. The second stage is per-

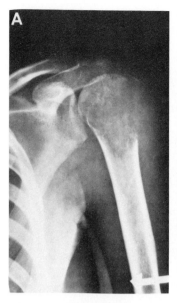

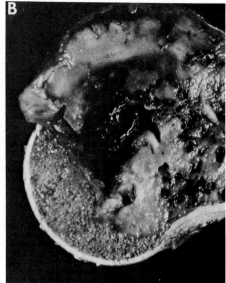

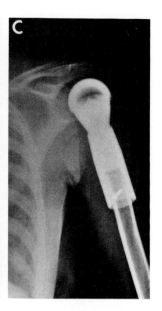

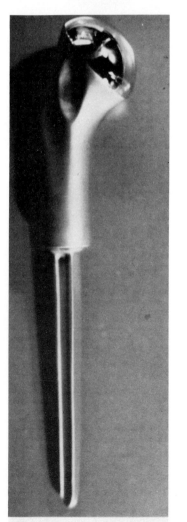

Fig. 8-12. *A*, Anteroposterior view of proximal humerus showing extensive destruction due to giant cell tumor. *B*, Surgical specimen after resection. *C*, After reconstruction with ceramic hemiarthroplasty.

Fig. 8-13. Custom Vitallium proximal humeral replacement prosthesis. Fixation is achieved by an intramedullary stem and methyl methacrylate.

formed 2 to 4 weeks later, with massive autogenous iliac grafts. Once these grafts have healed, the patient has a stable extremity that can withstand the forces required for normal daily activity (Fig. 8-16).

Clinical Material

Between 1970 and 1981, 102 of 285 patients with chondrosarcomas, 44 of 390 with osteosarcomas, and 14 of 75 with fibrosarcomas seen at the Mayo Clinic underwent limb-saving resection (Table 8-1). The average age was 37 years, and the average follow-up was 38 months. There were 75 males and 85 females.

All patients underwent extensive preoperative staging, which included plain radiographs, indicated laboratory tests, computed tomography of the chest (whole-lung tomography was used before 1975), computed tomography of the lesion, technetium bone scans, and arteriography in selected patients. The anatomic locations of the lesions are shown in Figure 8-17. No patients received adjuvant chemotherapy, which should allow a standard for comparison with centers doing these procedures under a protective blanket of chemotherapy.

We adopted the system advocated by Enneking et al (63) for staging musculoskeletal sarcomas, which has been outlined in Chapter 4. Although ours is a highly selected group of patients, this classification should allow accurate comparison with other series (Fig. 8-18). With this method, there were 42 patients with stage IA lesions, 51 with stage IB lesions, 8 with stage IIA lesions, and 59 with stage IIB lesions. We further divided each stage on the basis of pathologic diagnosis. Most of the chon-

Fig. 8-14. *A,* Illustration of technique of femoral iliac fusion after resection of osseous lesion in the pelvis. *B,* Anteroposterior view of left hip and hemipelvis showing chondrosarcoma involving the acetabular region. *C,* After resection of the chondrosarcoma and reconstruction with a femoral iliac arthrodesis.

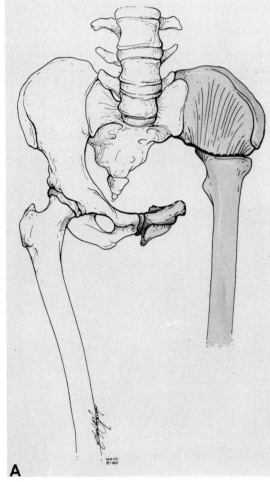

Fig. 8-14.

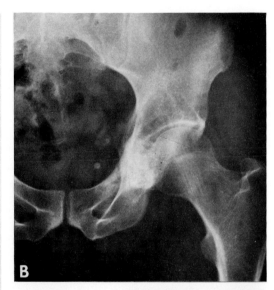

B

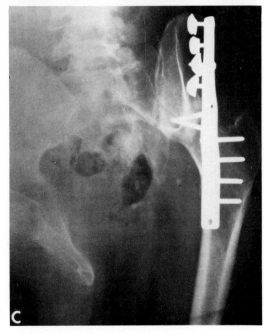

C

drosarcomas were low grade or stage IA and IB lesions. Most osteosarcomas, however, were high grade, with 27 patients having stage IIB. Also, most fibrosarcomas were high grade.

Surgical resection also was classified as recommended by Enneking et al (63) (see Chapter 4). With this method, 24 of the 42 patients with stage IA lesions underwent lesional or marginal resection; 44 of the 51 patients with stage IB lesions underwent wide resection; and 41 of the 59 patients with stage IIB lesions underwent wide resection. After resection, the method of reconstruction varied with the anatomic location of the tumor. In this series of 160 patients, 51 had no reconstruction, 49 had reconstruction with bone graft (allograft or autograft), and 60 had custom prosthetic reconstruction.

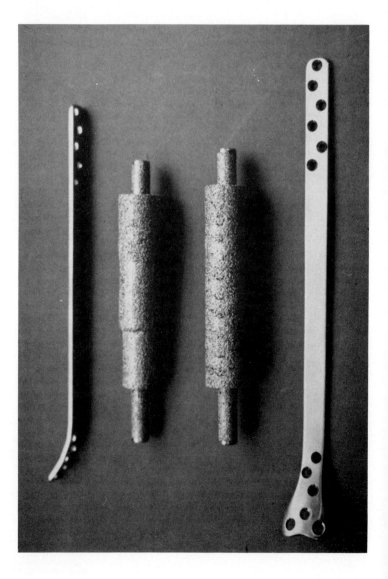

Fig. 8-15. Titanium fibermetal prosthesis used to reconstruct segmental defects in long bones after resection of tumors.

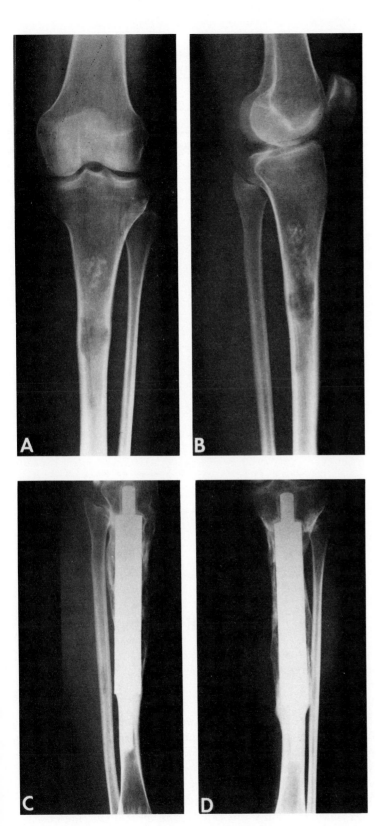

Fig. 8-16. Anteroposterior (*A*) and lateral (*B*) views of tibia showing an extensive grade 1 chondrosarcoma. Anteroposterior (*C*) and lateral (*D*) views of tibia after reconstruction utilizing a fibermetal prosthesis and autogenous bone grafts. The cortex has been reconstituted.

Table 8-1. Limb Salvage for Bone Sarcomas According to Surgical Stage (Mayo Clinic Series)

Pathologic diagnosis	Patients		Stage I		Stage II	
	No.	%	A	B	A	B
Chondrosarcoma	102	63.8	36	35	5	26
Osteosarcoma	44	27.5	4	13	0	27
Fibrosarcoma	14	8.7	2	3	3	6
Total	160	100.0	42	51	8	59

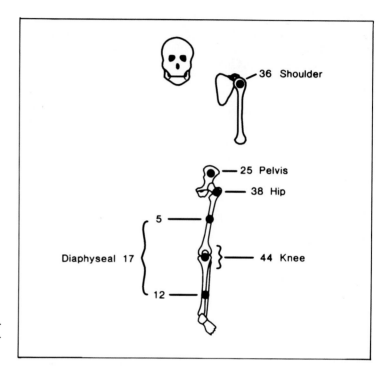

Fig. 8-17. Sites of primary malignant osseous lesions in patients treated with limb-salvage techniques.

Functional Results

Functional results were analyzed for each anatomic region and, when compared with the alternative of amputation, were far superior.

Proximal Femur. Of the 38 patients who underwent resection of malignant lesions of the proximal femur, 31 had custom prosthetic replacement (Fig. 8-19) (7 hemiarthroplasties, 24 total hip arthroplasties). The length of the segmental replacement varied from 80 to 250 mm. Functional results were evaluated by clinical examination and gait analysis.

A stable extremity was achieved in all patients, thereby allowing early mobilization and ambulation. Patients were ambulatory an average of 8.6 days (range 4 to 25 days) after surgical

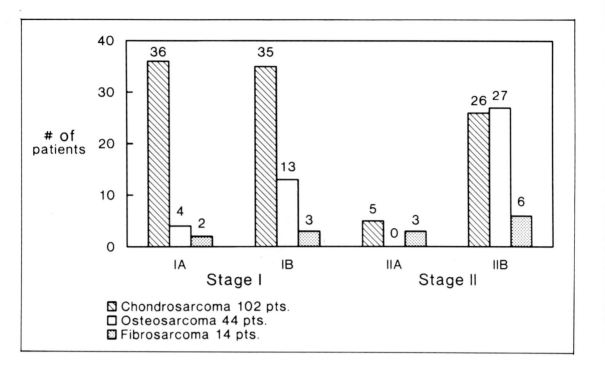

of
patients

40

30

20

10

0

36

35

26 27

13

4
2

5
0 3

6

3

IA   IB   IIA   IIB
Stage I   Stage II

◪ Chondrosarcoma 102 pts.
▢ Osteosarcoma 44 pts.
▩ Fibrosarcoma 14 pts.

Fig. 8-18. Surgical stages of bone sarcomas in patients undergoing limb-salvage procedures.

resection. All patients were able to ambulate independently. More than 70% of the patients had no complaints of pain at follow-up. Because the abductors were usually resected at surgery, we recommended that all of these patients use a cane when walking. Sixty-five percent of the patients used a single cane, while 18% used no support. Eighty-six percent of the patients had no limitation or had only mild limitation of activity.

Of the seven patients who did not undergo prosthetic reconstruction, two underwent reconstruction, one with an allograft and the other with autogenous bone grafts. The other five patients did not require reconstruction. Five of the seven patients had excellent functional results, one required a hemipelvectomy for local recurrence, and one died within 4 months of surgery.

Knee. Of the 44 patients with primary malignant tumors of the knee, 16 underwent prosthetic reconstruction (Fig. 8-20). The length of the replacement ranged from 76 to 180 mm. Functional results were evaluated in the same manner as was done for the patients with hip lesions.

Sixty-nine percent of the patients had no pain, and 31% had only mild pain. Eighty percent of the patients did not use walking aids, and the remainder used a single cane. Eighty-two percent had no limitations in activity. Knee motion averaged 85.2°. Of the remaining 28 patients, 11 required no reconstruction after resection. All 11 patients had excellent or good functional results, and none used walking aids. Of the 17 other patients, 11 had reconstruction with autogenous bone grafts, 5 had resection

Fig. 8-19. *A,* Anteroposterior view of right hip showing extensive stage IB chondrosarcoma. *B,* Surgical specimen after resection. *C,* Roentgenogram after resection and reconstruction with proximal femoral replacement.

arthrodesis, and 1 had an allograft. All 17 patients have excellent or good functional results, except for 1 patient who underwent resection arthrodesis and who developed a postoperative infection.

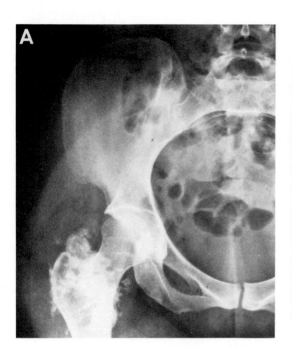

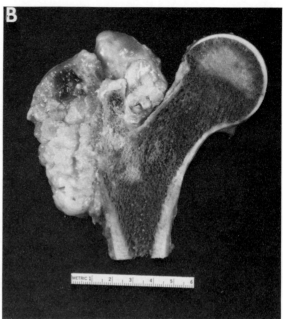

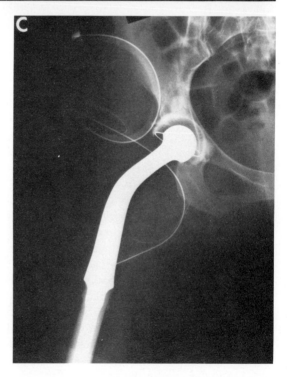

Bone Tumors

Shoulder. Because of the complex mechanics of the shoulder joint, the goal of reconstruction was to obtain normal hand and elbow function. In 10 patients, a prosthesis was used to act as a spacer after resection of the proximal humerus. Seven of these patients underwent reconstruction with a modular ceramic prosthesis fitted by extracortical cone fixation. The other three patients underwent reconstruction with a custom Vitallium prosthesis. Six of the patients had good results, and the remaining four had fair results.

Twelve patients needed no reconstruction. Seven of the 12 patients had a total or partial scapulectomy, two had a Tinkoff-Lindberg resection, and three underwent partial humeral resection. All 12 patients had excellent or good hand and elbow function.

Fourteen patients underwent reconstruction with autogenous grafts, and they also had excellent or good hand and elbow function.

Pelvis. Thirteen patients required no reconstruction, five required reconstruction with autogenous grafts, four had the femur fused to the remaining pelvis, and three were left with a flail femur. All of these patients had excellent or good functional results, except the three patients in whom the femur was left flail. All three of these patients had poor results.

Diaphyseal. Of the 17 patients with diaphyseal lesions, 5 underwent reconstruction with a titanium fibermetal prosthesis and autogenous bone grafts. Three of these patients had excellent results. Two had results that were considered satisfactory because they required a second operation for additional bone grafting.

Eleven patients had reconstruction—nine with autogenous bone grafts and two with allografts—and one patient required no reconstruction. All 12 of these patients had excellent or good results, except the 1 patient with an allograft, who developed an infection that required an amputation.

Complications, Local Recurrence, and Survival

Seven of the 160 patients developed infections (Table 8-2). In one patient, the infection did not resolve and amputation was required. In the prosthetic group, 4 of the 60 patients had loosening of the prosthesis which required revision. Three patients had fractures of the prosthesis which required revision, and 5 had dislocations of the prosthesis. The corrective procedures done for these patients were successful, with no subsequent complications at the time of follow-up.

Various prognostic factors were analyzed to determine their effects on local recurrence and survival. Age and sex were not

Limb Salvage and Reconstructive Techniques

significant. Although we continue to see patients in whom limb salvage is precluded by a poorly positioned biopsy site, in this series the time or the site of the biopsy seemed to have no effect on outcome.

Anatomic location was significant, in that more than 20% of patients with hip lesions had a local recurrence. However,

Table 8-2. Complications After Limb Salvage for Bone Sarcomas

Complication	Patient	
	No.	%
Infection*	7/160	4.4
Wound problems	5/160	3.1
Prosthetic problems		
Loosening	4/60	6.7
Fracture	3/60	5.0
Dislocation	5/60	8.3
Others	6/160	3.8
Tendon rupture	(1)	
Peroneal palsy	(1)	
Additional bone graft	(4)	

*One patient required amputation.

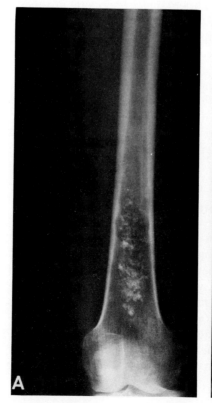

Fig. 8-20. *A,* Anteroposterior view of right distal femur showing a grade 1 chondrosarcoma that has dedifferentiated to a grade 4 osteosarcoma. *B,* After resection of the distal femur and reconstruction with a 200 mm Walldius total knee arthroplasty.

on further analysis, the more important factor seemed to be the surgical stage of the lesion; more than 70% of the patients with hip lesions had stage II or high-grade lesions (Fig. 8-21).

The differences among the rates of local recurrences for chondrosarcoma (11.8%), osteosarcoma (11.4%), and fibrosarcoma (14.3%) were not statistically significant. However, the average time for local recurrence to develop after resection was much longer with chondrosarcoma (40.6 months) than with osteosarcoma (7 months) or fibrosarcoma (14.5 months).

When the surgical stage was correlated with the surgical resection, only five of the local recurrences were seen in patients with stage I lesions. Fourteen of the 59 patients with stage IIB lesions had local recurrences, for a rate of 23.7%.

Limb salvage did not appear to affect survival adversely, with 84% of patients disease-free at an average follow-up of 38 months. Thirteen percent of the patients died or were alive with active disease. If the patient had a local recurrence, however, survival was adversely affected. Eight of the 19 patients with a local recurrence either had died or were alive with active disease at follow-up. Local recurrence was treated by amputation in 7 patients and by wide excision in 10 patients.

Histogenesis appeared to affect survival—only 2% of the patients with chondrosarcomas died compared to 24% of the patients with osteosarcomas and 14% of those with fibrosarcomas. Further analysis revealed that an important factor appeared to be the large number of high-grade osteosarcomas (62%) and fibrosarcomas (64%) compared with chondrosar-

Fig. 8-21. Recurrence rates and distribution of bone sarcomas according to stage and anatomic location in patients, undergoing limb-salvage procedures.

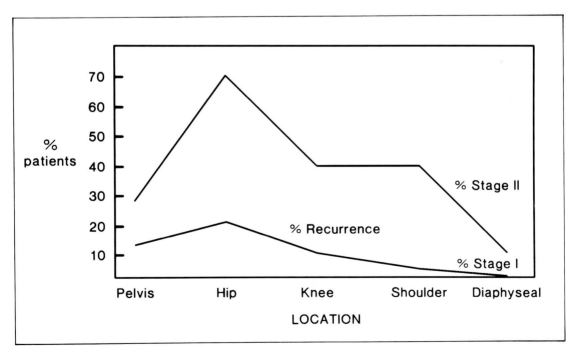

comas (30%). By 38 months, 12% of the patients with stage IIA lesions and 18% of those with stage IIB lesions had died, whereas only 2% and 4% of the patients with stage IA and IB lesions, respectively, had died.

Discussion

Considerable progress has been made in the treatment of primary malignant bone tumors. With recent projected 5-year survival rates of higher than 80%, enthusiasm for limb-sparing surgery is increasing rapidly (21). Whether this choice will prove to be a wise one remains to be seen. At the Mayo Clinic, we continue to be highly selective in recommending limb salvage, as is evidenced by the small percentage of our total patient population undergoing these procedures. We believe that, until more conclusive data exist, limb-sparing surgery should be considered experimental.

We have found the staging system advocated by Enneking et al (63) to be an accurate method of classifying each individual lesion. The need for such a system is obvious. It not only allows us to determine which patients may be suitable for limb salvage but also allows more meaningful comparisons of results among different institutions. We hope that all centers that treat large numbers of patients who have musculoskeletal tumors will use this method of classification.

Careful planning for the biopsy is very important. All preoperative studies should be completed before the biopsy specimen is taken. Transverse wounds on extremities should be avoided. Meticulous hemostasis should be obtained before a carefully layered closure of the incision is done. If the surgeon does not plan to perform the definitive surgery, the patient should be referred to a cancer treatment center before the biopsy is done. Although the time and the site of the biopsy had no effect on outcome in our series of 160 patients, we have seen many patients in whom a poorly positioned biopsy wound has precluded any chance of limb-sparing surgery.

The surgical resection of primary malignant tumors should follow the established principles of oncologic surgery. Whenever possible, the lesion should be resected with a normal cuff of tissue. If the margin of resection is compromised, amputation should be strongly considered. We strive to achieve a bony margin of 6 to 8 cm and a soft-tissue margin of at least 2 cm. When possible, we prefer to perform the reconstruction during the initial procedure. To achieve this goal, we maintain a large inventory of custom implants. The methods of reconstruction described are demanding and require meticulous attention to detail in order to avoid postoperative morbidity.

Each patient should be considered for limb salvage on an individual basis. The age of the patient is an important factor. Usually, amputation is the best treatment for a patient with open epiphyses. There have been reports of successful intercalary amputation in patients with high-grade malignancies about the knee (72). Although we have had no experience with this technique, functional results appear to be much better than with above-knee amputations. When limb salvage is technically possible in adolescents and young adults with malignant lesions of the knee, we prefer a resection arthrodesis over a custom implant because once healing is complete there is little risk of late failure.

The functional results of limb-sparing surgery have been gratifying when compared with the results after amputation, particularly those in the shoulder and the pelvis. The question that still remains unanswered concerns the long-term results of prosthetic reconstruction in the weight-bearing extremity. Our experience suggests that implant failure will continue and recovery will be very difficult. The new porous-coated prostheses, which allow bone ingrowth, may alleviate some of these problems, and further research should improve our armamentarium. The importance of a close liaison between the surgeon and the biomechanical engineer cannot be overemphasized.

In our series of 160 patients, the local recurrence rate of 23.7% in high-grade lesions is unacceptable. Other investigators are reporting much lower rates with the use of preoperative chemotherapy (14,19–21,72). Recently, we have begun a protocol of preoperative chemotherapy consisting of bleomycin, cisplatin, doxorubicin, and cyclophosphamide. Although we are uncertain of the value of adjunctive chemotherapy on improving survival, the use of preoperative chemotherapy may decrease the microscopic spread of tumor cells in the local area, thereby decreasing the local recurrence rate after resectional surgery.

Summary

Evaluation of limb salvage in a series of 160 patients indicates that, while these procedures are still experimental and more time is needed for follow-up, the early results promise utility and functional restoration. The Enneking staging system correlates well with prognosis and indicates that the surgical resection must be tailored to the surgical stage of the lesion. The high recurrence rate in patients with stage II lesions suggests the need for more effective surgical or adjuvant treatment.

References

1. Cade S: Osteogenic sarcoma: a study based on 133 patients. J R Coll Surg Edinb 1:79–111, 1955
2. Dahlin DC, Coventry MB: Osteogenic sarcoma: a study of six hundred cases. J Bone Joint Surg [Am] 49:101–110, 1967
3. Dahlin DC: Bone Tumors: General Aspects and Data on 6,221 Cases. Third edition. Springfield, Illinois, Charles C Thomas, Publisher, 1978
4. Enneking WF, Springfield DS: Osteosarcoma. Orthop Clin North Am 8:785–803, 1977
5. Ivins JC, Pritchard DJ: Management of osteogenic sarcoma at the Mayo Clinic. Recent Results Cancer Res 54:221–230, 1976

6. Sim FH, Ivins JC, Pritchard DJ: Surgical treatment of osteogenic sarcoma at the Mayo Clinic. Cancer Treat Res 62:205–211, 1978

7. Sweetnam R: The surgical management of primary osteosarcoma. Clin Orthop 111:57–64, 1975

8. Gitelis S, Bertoni F, Picci P, et al: Chondrosarcoma of bone: the experience at the Istituto Ortopedico Rizzoli. J Bone Joint Surg [Am] 63:1248–1257, 1981

9. Henderson ED, Dahlin DC: Chondrosarcoma of bone—a study of two hundred and eighty-eight cases. J Bone Joint Surg [Am] 45:1450–1458, 1963

10. Marcove RC, Miké V, Hutter RVP, et al: Chondrosarcoma of the pelvis and upper end of the femur: an analysis of factors influencing survival time in one hundred and thirteen cases. J Bone Joint Surg [Am] 54:561–572, 1972

11. Pritchard DJ, Lunke RJ, Taylor WF, et al: Chondrosarcoma: a clinicopathologic and statistical analysis. Cancer 45:149–157, 1980

12. Smith WS, Simon MA: Segmental resection for chondrosarcoma. J Bone Joint Surg [Am] 57:1097–1103, 1975

13. Bowden L, Booher RJ: The principles and technique of resection of soft parts for sarcoma. Surgery 44:963–977, 1958

14. Eilber FR, Mirra JJ, Grant TT, et al: Is amputation necessary for sarcomas? A seven-year experience with limb salvage. Ann Surg 192:431–437, 1980

15. Phemister DB: Conservative surgery in the treatment of bone tumors. Surg Gynecol Obstet 70:355–364, 1940

16. Campanacci M, Bacci G, Bertoni F, et al: The treatment of osteosarcoma of the extremities: twenty years' experience at the Istituto Ortopedico Rizzoli. Cancer 48:1569–1581, 1981

17. Edmonson JH, Green SJ, Ivins JC, et al: Methotrexate as adjuvant treatment for primary osteosarcoma. N Engl J Med 303:642–643, 1980

18. Gilchrist GS, Pritchard DJ, Dahlin DC, et al: Management of osteogenic sarcoma: a perspective based on the Mayo Clinic experience. Natl Cancer Inst Monogr 56:193–199, 1981

19. Jaffe N, Watts H, Fellows KE, et al: Local en bloc resection for limb preservation. Cancer Treat Rep 62:217–223, 1978

20. Marcove RC, Rosen G: En bloc resections for osteogenic sarcoma. Cancer 45:3040–3044, 1980

21. Rosen G, Caparros B, Huvos AG, et al: Preoperative chemotherapy for osteogenic sarcoma: selection of postoperative adjuvant chemotherapy based on the response of the primary tumor to preoperative chemotherapy. Cancer 49:1221–1230, 1982

22. Bleyer WA, Haas JE, Feigl P, et al: Improved three-year disease-free survival in osteogenic sarcoma. J Bone Joint Surg [Br] 64:233–238, 1982

23. Cortes EP, Holland JF, Wang JJ, et al: Amputation and adriamycin in primary osteosarcoma. N Engl J Med 291:998–1000, 1974

24. Jaffe N, Frei E III, Traggis D, et al: Adjuvant methotrexate and citrovorum-factor treatment of osteogenic sarcoma. N Engl J Med 291:994–997, 1974

25. Jaffe N: Osteogenic sarcoma: state of the art with high-dose methotrexate treatment. Clin Orthop 120:95–102, 1976

26. Marcove RC: En bloc resections for osteogenic sarcoma. Cancer Treat Rep 62:225–231, 1978

27. Rosen G, Marcove RC, Caparros B, et al: Primary osteogenic sarcoma: the rationale for preoperative chemotherapy and delayed surgery. Cancer 43:2163–2177, 1979

28. Schajowicz F: Juxtacortical chondrosarcoma. J Bone Joint Surg [Br] 59:473–480, 1977

29. Taylor WF, Ivins JC, Dahlin DC, et al: Trends and variability in survival from osteosarcoma. Mayo Clin Proc 53:695–700, 1978

30. Unni KK, Dahlin DC, Beabout JW: Periosteal osteogenic sarcoma. Cancer 37:2476–2485, 1976

31. Unni KK, Dahlin DC, Beabout JW, et al: Parosteal osteogenic sarcoma. Cancer 37:2466–2475, 1976
32. Unni KK, Dahlin DC, McLeod RA, et al: Intraosseous well-differentiated osteosarcoma. Cancer 40:1337–1347, 1977
33. Campanacci M, Costa P: Total resection of distal femur or proximal tibia for bone tumours: autogenous bone grafts and arthrodesis in twenty-six cases. J Bone Joint Surg [Br] 61:455–463, 1979
34. Dobbs HS, Scales JT, Wilson JN, et al: Endoprosthetic replacement of the proximal femur and acetabulum: a survival analysis. J Bone Joint Surg [Br] 63:219–224, 1981
35. Johnston JO: Local resection in primary malignant bone tumors. Clin Orthop 153:73–80, 1980
36. Koskinen EVS, Salenius P, Alho A: Allogeneic transplantation in low-grade malignant bone tumours: a new operative technique to avoid amputation. Acta Orthop Scand 50:129–138, 1979
37. Sim FH, Pritchard DJ, Ivins JC, et al: Total joint arthroplasty: applications in the management of bone tumors. Mayo Clin Proc 54:583–589, 1979
38. Watts HG: Introduction to resection of musculoskeletal sarcomas. Clin Orthop 153:31–38, 1980
39. Eiselsberg AF: Zur Heilung Grösserer Defecte der Tibia durch gestielte Haute-Periost-Knochenlappen. Arch Klin Chir 55:435–444, 1897
40. Klapp R: Ueber einen Fall von ausgedehnter Knochentransplantation. Deutsche Ztschr Chir 54:576–583, 1900
41. Albee FH: The treatment of primary malignant changes of the bone: by radical resection with bone graft replacement. JAMA 107:1693–1698, 1936
42. Phemister DB: Rapid repair of defect of femur by massive bone grafts after resection for tumors. Surg Gynecol Obstet 80:120–127, 1945
43. Coley BL, Higinbotham NL: Conservative surgery in tumors of bone: with special reference to segmental resection. Ann Surg 127:231–242, 1948
44. Coley BL, Higinbotham NL: Giant-cell tumor of bone. J Bone Joint Surg 20:870–884, 1938
45. Inclan A, Leon P: The result of primary block resection in bone tumors. South Med J 46:537–544, 1953
46. Johnson EW Jr, Dahlin DC: Treatment of giant-cell tumor of bone. J Bone Joint Surg [Am] 41:895–904, 1959
47. Lexer E: Joint transplantations and arthroplasty. Surg Gynecol Obstet 40:782–809, 1925
48. Judet: Cited by Lexer E (47)
49. Parrish FF: Allograft replacement of all or part of the end of a long bone following excision of a tumor: report of twenty-one cases. J Bone Joint Surg [Am] 55:1–22, 1973
50. Parrish FF: Treatment of bone tumors by total excision and replacement with massive autologous and homologous grafts. J Bone Joint Surg [Am] 48:968–990, 1966
51. Mankin HJ, Fogelson FS, Thrasher AZ, et al: Massive resection and allograft transplantation in the treatment of malignant bone tumors. N Engl J Med 294:1247–1255, 1976
52. Hiki Y, Mankin HJ: Radical resection and allograft replacement in the treatment of bone tumors. Nippon Seikeigeka Gakkai Zasshi 54:475, 1980
53. Eilber FA: Personal communication.
54. Merle d'Aubigné R, Dejouany JP: Diaphyso-epiphysial resection for bone tumour at the knee: with reports of nine cases. J Bone Joint Surg [Br] 40:385–395, 1958
55. Wilson PD, Lance EM: Surgical reconstruction of the skeleton following segmental resection for bone tumors. J Bone Joint Surg [Am] 47:1629–1656, 1965
56. Enneking WF, Shirley PD: Resection-arthrodesis for malignant and

potentially malignant lesions about the knee using an intramedullary rod and local bone grafts. J Bone Joint Surg [Am] 59:223–236, 1977

57. Moore AT, Bohlman HR: Metal hip joint: a case report. J Bone Joint Surg 25:688–692, 1943

58. Kraft GL, Levinthal DH: Acrylic prosthesis replacing lower end of the femur for benign giant-cell tumor. J Bone Joint Surg [Am] 36:368–374, 1954

59. Burrows HJ, Wilson JN, Scales JT: Excision of tumours of humerus and femur, with restoration by internal prostheses. J Bone Joint Surg [Br] 57:148–159, 1975

60. Marcove RC, Lewis MM, Rosen G, et al: Total femur and total knee replacement: a preliminary report. Clin Orthop 126:147—152, 1977

61. Sim FH, Chao EY, Peterson LFA: Reconstruction following segmental resection of primary bone tumors of the hip. Hip 3:302–324, 1975

62. Volkov M: Allotransplantation of joints. J Bone Joint Surg [Br] 52:49–53, 1970

63. Enneking WF, Spanier SS, Goodman MA: A system for the surgical staging of musculoskeletal sarcoma. Clin Orthop 153:106–120, 1980

64. Galante J, Rostoker W, Luecke R, et al: Sintered fiber metal composites as a basis for attachment of implants to bone. J Bone Joint Surg [Am] 53:101–114, 1971

65. Kotz R, Salzer M: Resection therapy of malignant tumours of the shoulder girdle. Osterr Z Onkol 2:97–109, 1975

66. Enneking WF: Personal communication

67. Enneking WF, Dunham WK: Resection and reconstruction for primary neoplasms involving the innominate bone. J Bone Joint Surg [Am] 60:731–746, 1978

68. Johnson JTH: Reconstruction of the pelvic ring following tumor resection. J Bone Joint Surg [Am] 60:747–751, 1978

69. Steel HH: Partial or complete resection of the hemipelvis: an alternative to hindquarter amputation for periacetabular chondrosarcoma of the pelvis. J Bone Joint Surg [Am] 60:719–730, 1978

70. Zatsepin ST: Conservative operations for pelvic bone tumours. Int Orthop 4:259–268, 1981

71. Mankin HJ: Personal communication

72. Salzer M, Knahr K, Kotz R, et al: Treatment of osteosarcomata of the distal femur by rotation-plasty. Arch Orthop Trauma Surg 99:131–136, 1982

Section II:

Benign Tumors

CHAPTER 9

BENIGN TUMORS

Franklin H. Sim, M.D.
Krishnan K. Unni, M.B., B.S.
Lester E. Wold, M.D.
Richard A. McLeod, M.D.

The classification of bone tumors which is used by most surgical pathologists is based on the histologic appearance of the tissue produced by the cells (1). Benign tumors of bone may arise from several histologic types—chondrogenic, osteogenic, and fibrogenic—as well as from the main components of normal bone; but they may also arise from vascular, neurogenic, or lipogenic elements or they may even be of unknown origin. The conditions that simulate bone tumors also must be considered because they cause equal concern and difficulty, both in diagnosis and treatment. Of the 6,221 primary bone tumors in the files of the Mayo Clinic, 1,447 were benign bone tumors.

Tumors of Chondrogenic Origin

Osteochondroma   (Osteocartilaginous Exostosis)
Osteochondroma is the most common benign bone tumor, accounting for 40% of the benign lesions in the Mayo Clinic series (2) (Fig. 9-1). However, the incidence is actually higher because most of the patients are asymptomatic and the tumors are not removed. These lesions occur more commonly in males. The tumor begins in childhood and continues to grow until skeletal maturity is reached. In the Mayo Clinic series, approximately 60% of the patients were less than 20 years of age when the lesion was removed.

The tumor occurs in any bone but usually develops in the

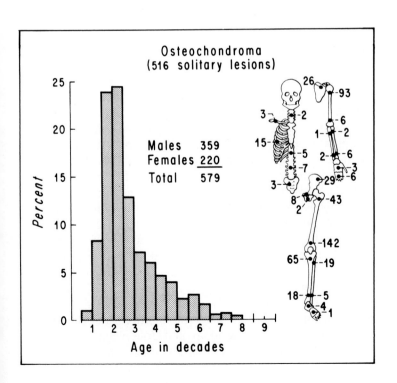

9-1. Age and sex incidence of pa-
; with osteochondroma, Mayo Clinic
rience. (From Dahlin DC: Bone Tu-
: General Aspects and Data on 6,221
's. Third edition. Springfield, Illinois,
les C Thomas, 1978, p 18. By per-
on.)

metaphyseal region of the long bones, particularly the distal femur, and enlarges by progressive endochondral ossification of a growing cartilagenous cap. The cap is attached to a bony stalk (pedunculated) or to a broad base of bone (Fig. 9-3 *A*). On roentgenographic examination, the bony stalk may be seen projecting from the surface of the bone, usually away from the adjacent joint (Fig. 9-2 *A*). On the roentgenogram, the lesion appears to be smaller than it actually is, because the cartilage component is not well seen. Evidence of calcification may be seen within a cartilage cap, and if the cartilage cap appears to be large, the possibility of sarcomatous change should be considered. We have treated 22 patients who had solitary exostosis that gave rise to chondrosarcomas. This, of course, is a selected series, as the 4.1% incidence of malignant change actually indicates that less than 1% of solitary osteochondromas subsequently become malignant. Roentgenographically, the periosteal surface and the cortex of the tumor are contiguous with the underlying bone, as is the medullary cavity, which may contain either fatty or hematopoietic marrow. Most osteochondromas have a smooth cartilaginous cap, 2 to 3 mm in thickness. The lesion should be cut perpendicular to the cartilaginous cap. If the cap is irregular or greater than 2 cm thick, then careful histologic study of the tissue is warranted because of the possibility of secondary chondrosarcoma (1).

Microscopically, the cartilaginous cap of an osteochondroma is characterized by mature chondrocytes arranged in a single-file pattern that mimics the appearance of normal epiphyseal cartilage. There is an associated region of enchondral ossification, with fatty or hematopoietic marrow between the trabeculae (Fig. 9-3 *B*). Fibroblastic proliferation and accompanying new bone formation may be seen secondary to trauma.

Routine removal of these tumors is not justified unless the lesion is large enough to cause symptoms from mechanical irritation or is growing disproportionately in size. Occasionally, the lesion is removed for cosmetic reasons. When necessary, adequate removal involves thorough excision of the base of the exostosis, with care being taken to remove the entire cartilage cap, and this is nearly always curative (Fig. 9-2 *B*). Occasionally, excision requires a bone graft if the base is broad and the bone is weakened when the exostosis is removed (Fig. 9-2 *C*). A patient may have multiple osteochondromas, and when present, these involve many different bones and may produce a dysplastic appearance of the involved bones. Each individual tumor has characteristics described for the solitary lesion. These lesions have a higher risk of developing sarcomatous change, probably about 10%. While the harvesting of all these lesions is not indicated, patients with multiple osteochondromas need to be carefully followed up, and large symptomatic lesions that are changing should be excised with a marginal or wide margin.

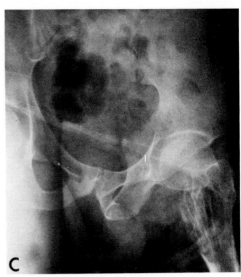

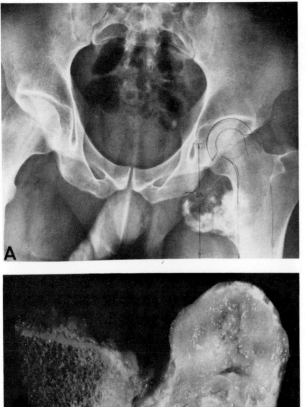

Fig. 9-2. *A*, Anteroposterior view of pelvis and proximal femur showing large osteochondroma in lesser trochanteric region. Thick, irregular cartilage cap was worrisome for secondary malignancy. *B*, Excised specimen with underlying margin of normal bone. *C*, After insertion of autogenous bone grafts to defect.

Chondroma. Chondroma is a lesion of mature hyaline cartilage occurring either centrally in the bone (enchondroma) (Fig. 9-4) or, less frequently, in the periosteum (periosteal or cortical chondroma). These lesions composed 11.2% of the benign tumors in the Mayo Clinic series (1) and occurred without significant sex predilection (Fig. 9-5). The lesion may be found at any age and in virtually any bone. More than 40% of the tumors occur in the hands (2) and feet, and approximately 90% of these occur in the hands. Since the lesion consists of mature hyaline cartilage, it grows very slowly and is usually asymptomatic. Often, the enchondroma is discovered fortuitously on roentgenograms performed for unrelated conditions. Any pain that occurs with the tumor is usually associated with a pathologic fracture. In the absence of a fracture, pain is suggestive of the possibility of malignancy. Occasionally, a painless swelling is the first manifestation, especially in the hand, giving the phalanx or the metacarpal a fusiform appearance (3).

Grossly, the lesion is composed of lobulated masses of bluish, semitranslucent hyaline cartilage. Calcification may occasionally be appreciated grossly and results in the characteristic punctate calcific deposits that are seen on the roentgenogram. Microscopically, chondroma is characterized by lobules of hyaline cartilage (Fig. 9-6). The chondrocytes lie within lacunae and have small nuclei. The cellularity of the tumors varies considerably from tumor to tumor and from one area within a tumor to another. Occasional binucleated chondrocytes may be seen; however, multinucleated chondrocytes and cells with large nuclei should alert the pathologist that the lesion may be malignant.

The microscopic differentiation of a chondroma from a low-grade chondrosarcoma may be extremely difficult. The location of the tumor and the presence or absence of roentgenographic evidence of endosteal erosion are very helpful. Hypercellular lesions with enlarged and binucleated cells occurring in the small bones of the hands and feet, and with a roentgenographic appearance suggesting benignancy, may be safely considered to be benign, whereas a similar tumor located in the pelvis, shoulder girdle, or rib probably will behave in a low-grade malignant fashion. The presence of endosteal erosion also should alert the pathologist to the presence of a low-grade chondrosarcoma.

The periosteal chondroma is characterized by a well-demarcated, saucer-shaped erosion of the underlying bone with extension into the surrounding soft tissues (4, 5) (Fig. 9-7). The medullary cavity of the underlying bone is not involved. Microscopically, the tumor may exhibit an alarming degree of hypercellularity and cellular atypia. However, if the radiographic appearance is consistent with a benign lesion, then these features do not indicate malignancy.

Rarely, the patient may have evidence of multiple chondromas, and when there is widespread involvement and an element of dysplasia, the condition is referred to as Ollier's disease; this

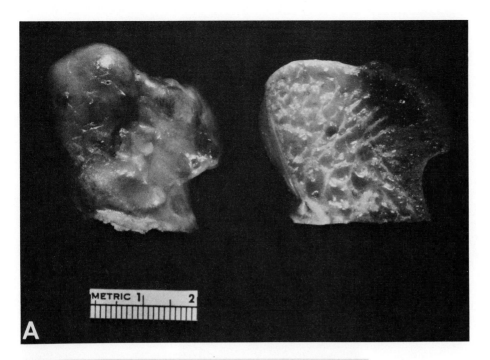

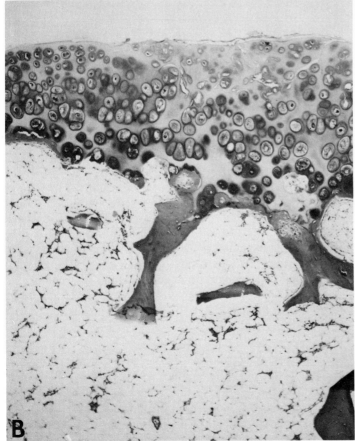

Fig. 9-3. *A*, Thin cartilaginous cap and lobulated gross appearance are typical of osteochondroma. Fatty marrow can be identified grossly beneath cap. *B*, Thin cartilaginous cap associated with enchondral ossification. Fatty marrow is noted between bony trabeculae. (Hematoxylin and eosin; x64.)

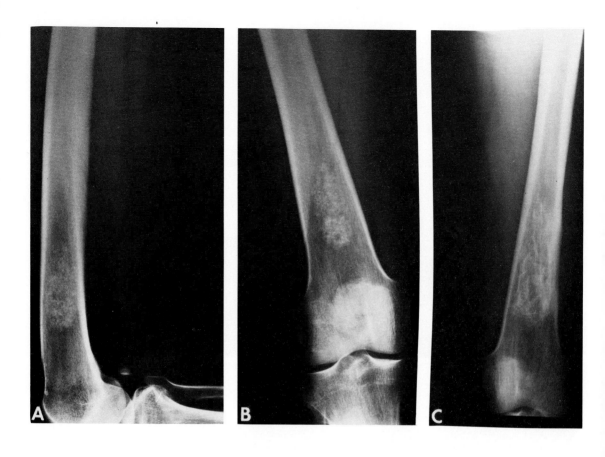

Fig. 9-4. Lateral (*A*) and anteroposterior (*B*) views of distal femur showing benign central cartilage lesion. *C*, After excision by curettage and bone grafting.

was present in 26 patients in the Mayo Clinic series (1). In the initial description of this syndrome, there was a tendency to unilaterality. This disease represents a failure of normal endochondral ossification. When there is evidence of multiple chondromas associated with angiomas of the soft tissue, the condition is referred to as Maffucci's syndrome (6).

Microscopic examination of the lesion in multiple chondromas shows hypercellular zones (more evident in younger patients) that resemble low-grade chondrosarcoma (6). Hypercellularity or zones of myxoid change should not dissuade the pathologist from making a diagnosis of benignity if the roentgenographic appearance of the tumors is suggestive of Ollier's dyschondroplasia.

Roentgenographically, an enchondroma appears as a well-marginated zone of lysis which frequently contains stippled calcification. This calcification usually is more prominent when the lesion occurs in long bones. Enchondromas of the hands and feet are rarely worrisome of malignancy. When a large lesion occurs in a large bone, it may be difficult by clinical examination and on the roentgenogram to determine whether the lesion is benign or is a low-grade chondrosarcoma. The presence of a

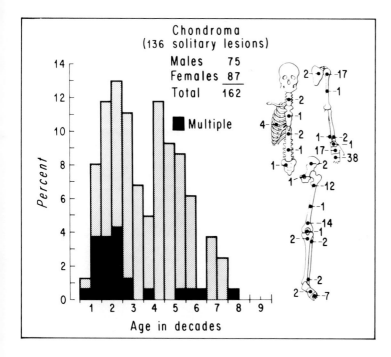

Fig. 9-5. Age and sex distribution of patients with chondroma, Mayo Clinic experience. (From Dahlin DC: Bone Tumors: General Aspects and Data on 6,221 Cases. Third edition. Springfield, Illinois, Charles C Thomas, 1978, p 29. By permission.)

pathologic fracture, scalloping of the endosteal cortical bone, or lytic areas in a mineralized lesion is suspicious for malignancy.

While surgical intervention is the preferred treatment, this must be dictated by the circumstances. Observation may be recommended when there is a benign-appearing small asymptomatic lesion that does not structurally weaken the bone, particularly in a young patient. Curettage is the treatment of choice for most patients with enchondromas. We also use adjuvant chemical cauterization, and bone grafts are usually necessary to restore the architecture of the bone; in an expendable small bone such as a rib or fibula, resection is preferred. With an associated pathologic fracture, this procedure is best done after the fracture has healed and the continuity of the bone has been restored. A periosteal chondroma (Fig. 9-8) may be confused with a chondrosarcoma, and patients with the former lesion are best treated by en bloc resection (5). The prognosis for the patient with a chondroma treated in this manner is good, and recurrence is not common; however, the lesion can recur if it was not completely excised. In addition, in many cases, lesions that have been described as recurrent chondromas are later found to have been originally underdiagnosed. Therefore, after recurrence, these lesions often appear to be more anaplastic than the original lesions. However, malignant transformation of a solitary chondroma probably is extremely rare.

Much concern is seen with a borderline cartilage tumor when the lesion presents with the typical radiographic and histologic findings of either an active chondroma or a low-grade chondro-

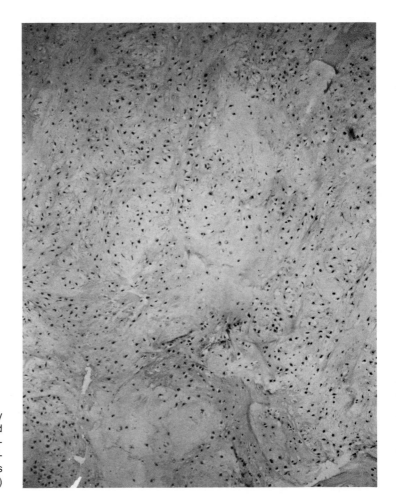

Fig. 9-6. Chondroma characterized by hypercellular chondroid matrix occurred in finger. This type of lesion most commonly has a benign-appearing radiographic appearance in spite of its cellularity. (Hematoxylin and eosin; x64.)

Fig. 9-7. *A*, Anteroposterior view showing periosteal chondroma in right proximal femur. *B*, Surgical specimen showing typical translucent hyaline cartilage.

sarcoma. It is particularly ominous if the patient presents with pain. In these lesions, it is probably best to achieve a marginal or wide margin by excision or resection. This, however, causes considerable loss of function and requires reconstruction of the segmental defect by autogenous or allograft bone. We have treated a number of patients with borderline lesions by radical exteriorization excision curettage, cauterization, and bone grafting. However, these patients need to be followed up for a long time because such lesions may recur years after the original treatment.

Benign Chondroblastoma. Benign chondroblastoma is a rare tumor in which the basic proliferating cells are remarkably similar to those of a true giant cell tumor but produce a chondroid matrix. First called "calcifying giant cell tumor" by Ewing (7) in 1928, then "epiphyseal chondromatous giant cell tumor" by Codman (8) in 1931, and finally "benign chondroblastoma" by Jaffe and Lichtenstein (9) in 1942, this lesion is usually found in the epiphysis of a long bone in the immature skeleton and it

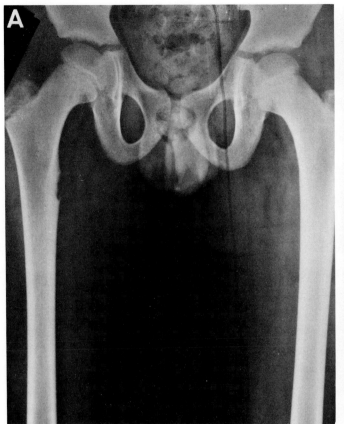
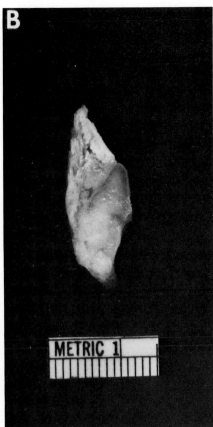

Fig. 9-7.

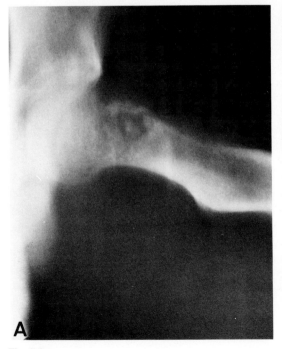
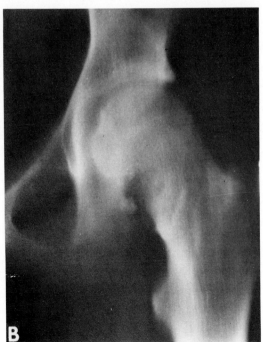

Fig. 9-8.

Benign Tumors

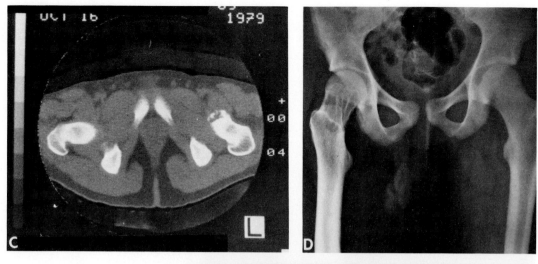

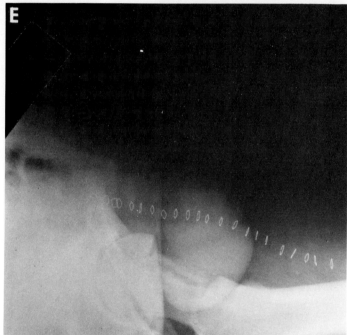

Fig. 9-8. Lateral (*A*) and anteroposterior (*B*) tomograms of right hip showing periosteal chondroma in femoral neck. Cortical irregularity and mineralization are worrisome for malignancy. *C*, Computed tomogram showing extent of lesion and destructive nature of cortex. Anteroposterior (*D*) and lateral (*E*) views of hip after excision and bone grafting.

can occur in a wide variety of bones (10). When this lesion occurs in adults, it is frequently in an unusual site, for example, innominate bone or scapula.

The tumor accounted for less than 1% of the Mayo Clinic series on bone tumors (11) (Fig. 9-9) and is approximately one-sixth as common as giant cell tumor. More than half of the patients are males, and most of the patients are in the second

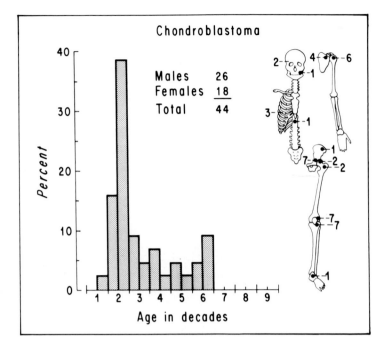

Fig. 9-9. Age and sex incidence of patients with chondroblastoma, Mayo Clinic experience. (From Dahlin DC: Bone Tumors: General Aspects and Data on 6,221 Cases. Third edition. Springfield, Illinois, Charles C Thomas, 1978, p 43. By permission.)

decade when the lesion is diagnosed. Local pain is an almost constant finding and is often referred to the adjacent joint.

Examination may reveal local wasting and, rarely, effusion in the adjacent joint. This has led to an erroneous diagnosis of joint disease in some cases. Radiographically, there is usually a central region of bone destruction involved in the epiphysis, at times with metaphyseal extension, usually while the growth plate is still open (Fig. 9-10). The lesion may be eccentric, with bulging expansion of the overlying cortex. Frequently, there is a sclerotic margin that delineates the lesion from the surrounding normal bone. About 25% show areas of matrix calcification within the radiolucent zone.

Grossly, the lesion is grayish pink and may contain zones of hemorrhage or necrosis (Fig. 9-11 *A*). Curetted fragments of tumor may contain chondroid flecks or whitish calcified material.

Microscopically, the tumor is characterized by a sheetlike proliferation of mononuclear cells (Fig. 9-11 *B*). The cells have abundant pinkish cytoplasm with distinct cytoplasmic boundaries between the cells. The nuclei of these cells often have a longitudinal groove, similar to that in the histiocytes of histiocytosis X. Scattered within the proliferating mononuclear cells are multinucleated giant cells and chondroid islands. The chondroid zones may be prominent or rare, and calcification frequently occurs within them.

Recognition of this entity is important clinically in that it is relatively nonaggressive and relatively curable, compared with giant cell tumor. The usual chondroblastoma is best treated by

Benign Tumors

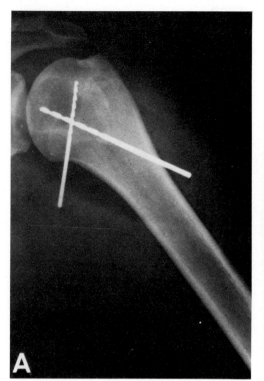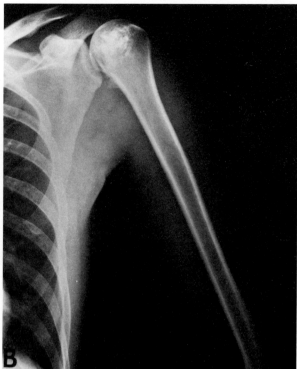

Fig. 9-10. *A*, Interoperative roentgeno-gram showing localization of typical chon-droblastoma in proximal humerus. *B*, After curettage and bone grafting.

curettage and bone grafting. The surgical approach and exter-iorization must be planned so as to preserve the growth plate if possible (Fig. 9-12). The optimal situation is when the chon-droblastoma is so located that it can be completely excised with the surrounding shell of normal bone, without significantly com-promising the function of the neighboring joint.

Cryosurgery has been advocated by some surgeons. The prognosis after treatment is excellent. There have been no re-currences in the Mayo Clinic series of 44 patients (11). Rarely, the presence of pulmonary metastasis in benign chondroblas-toma has been reported, but the metastatic lesions, like those of benign giant cell tumors, which metastasize to the lungs, tend to be nonprogressive and are usually not lifethreatening. Ra-diation for the primary lesion is to be avoided because of the chance for malignant transformation.

Chondromyxoid Fibroma. Chondromyxoid fibroma is the least common benign tumor of cartilage derivation and accounted for only half of 1% of the bone tumors in the Mayo Clinic series (1) (Fig. 9-13). As in most other bone tumors, a definite pre-dilection for males was found; most of the patients were in their second and third decades. The lesion is most often located in the metaphyseal region, usually near the epiphysis, and radi-ographically, it is most often seen as an eccentric, well-circumscribed rarefaction with sclerotic scalloped margins (Fig. 9-14). Approximately two-thirds of the lesions occur in long tubular bones, with approximately one-third being in the tibia. Chondromyxoid fibroma in a small bone can produce fusiform expansion. The roentgenographic features of this lesion are consistently those of a benign tumor (Fig. 9-15). A pathologic fracture occurred in 4 of the 30 patients in the Mayo Clinic series (1). The tumor is usually small, varying up to 5 cm in diameter.

Grossly, the tumor is firm and lobulated. The tumor is well circumscribed, has a benign roentgenographic appearance, and has a distinctly lobulated gross appearance (Fig. 9-15).

Microscopically, the hallmark of this tumor is its lobulated pattern (Fig. 9-16). The central portion of the tumor lobule is hypocellular, and the stellate and spindle cells are condensed at the periphery. The fibroma is myxoid, and only very rarely is true cartilage found. Phagocytic mononuclear cells, as well as giant cells, may be noted between the tumor lobules. The microscopic fields may be indistinguishable from those of chondroblastoma, and this suggests that the lesions have a common cell of origin.

Excision of the lesion is the treatment of choice (12). Curettage with grafting, although ordinarily successful, has a risk of recurrence of approximately 15%. When feasible, en bloc excision designed to include a margin of normal bone is preferable (3). Radiation therapy is not indicated, except for the rare inaccessible tumor. In the Mayo Clinic series (1), two patients underwent amputation, another patient with an extremely large tumor required amputation, and two patients with metatarsal tumors had ray resections.

Tumors of Osteogenic Origin

Osteoid Osteoma. Osteoid osteoma is a peculiar small benign bone tumor. Since first described by Jaffe (13) in 1935, it has become a well-recognized clinical and pathologic entity (14). The clinical pattern is characteristic, the radiologic features are usually distinctive, and the pathologic findings are unmistakable.

In the Mayo Clinic series (1), 158 osteomas composed 11% of the benign tumors (Fig. 9-17). There was a pronounced predominance of males. Ninety percent of the lesions occurred in patients who were 5 to 20 years old. The lesion was most frequent in the femur and tibia, but it can be found in any bone and is usually less than 1 cm in diameter.

The patient complains of unremitting and gradually increasing pain; night pain is particularly prominent. Aspirin seems to be specific for the pain, with most patients noting dramatic relief when given low doses of salicylates. Recent studies indicate increased levels of prostaglandins in patients with these lesions, and prostaglandin inhibitors have been noted to give relief. Pain is often experienced at a site remote from the lesion; for example, a lesion in the proximal femur may cause pain in the knee. Another peculiar feature is that the lesion may be associated with localized atrophy. This clinical syndrome of referred pain and atrophy often leads to an erroneous neurologic diagnosis.

We reviewed a series of 35 patients who presented with lumbar disk syndrome caused by a bone tumor in the spinal column or pelvis (15). Of these patients, approximately half had had disk surgery and the other half had had myelography before the true nature of the problem was discovered. It is very common for an osteoid osteoma of the spinal column or pelvis to mimic a lumbar disk syndrome. Moreover, the lesion may masquerade as idiopathic scoliosis. In this situation, the main clue to its true nature may be a worsening of the scoliosis when the supine position is assumed.

The essential part of this tumor is the nidus, which grossly is usually pinkish, granular, and distinct from the reactive surrounding sclerotic bone (Fig. 9-18 A). The nidus is usually soft enough to be cut on frozen section and need not be decalcified

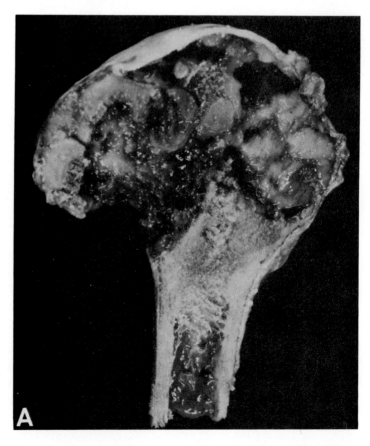

Fig. 9-11. A, Chondroblastoma of upper humerus. Resection of tumor was undertaken after recurrence. Tumor extended through cortex and to articular surface. B, Sheetlike proliferation of mononuclear cells and scattered multinucleated giant cells. Chondroid zones are variably present. (Hematoxylin and eosin: x250.)

before being embedded in paraffin. When the nidus is sclerotic, it is hardest near the center of the tumor. Radiographic guidance occasionally may be helpful in locating the nidus in the excised specimen.

The nidus of the tumor is composed of a tightly woven mass of osteoid trabeculae rimmed by osteoblasts (Fig. 9-18 B). The nidus is distinctly demarcated from the surrounding sclerotic bone. The osteoid trabeculae of the nidus are usually thin and variably mineralized. Between the bony trabeculae, there is loose fibrovascular connective tissue, within which multinucleated giant cells may be seen.

Often the lesion is obscure, and considerable skill is needed to demonstrate the lesion roentgenographically, after it has become suspected on the basis of the characteristic history (Fig. 9-19). When a clinical situation suggests the possibility of an osteoid osteoma, plain roentgenograms are usually obtained. In approximately 75% of the cases, the lesion can be confidently diagnosed on the roentgenogram. The main clue is a small radiolucent nidus, which is often located within the cortex of the bone. In this location, the nidus is usually surrounded by reactive sclerosis and dense periosteal new bone (Fig. 9-20 A and

Fig. 9-11.

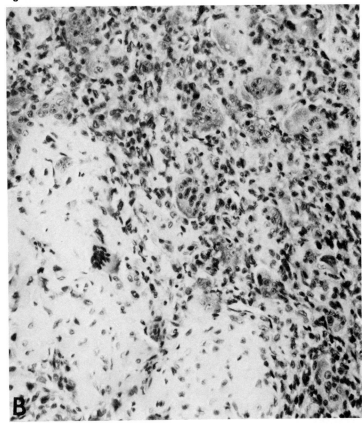

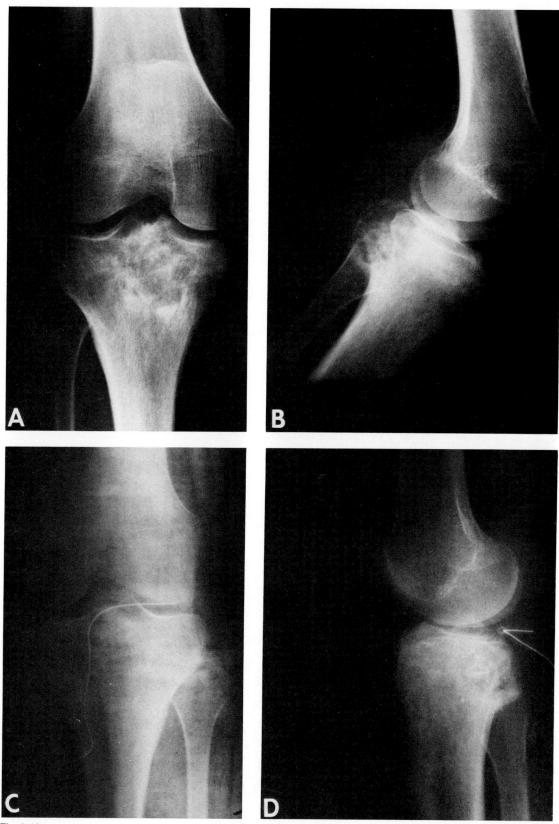

Fig. 9-12.

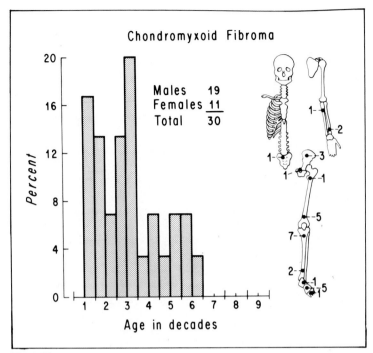

Fig. 9-13.

Fig. 9-12. Anteroposterior (*A*) and lateral (*B*) views of knee showing verified lesion of proximal tibia situated posteriorly and extending to the articular surface. Flecks of calcium are present in this benign chondroblastoma. *C* and *D*, After curettage and bone grafting.

Fig. 9-13. Age and sex incidence of patients with chondromyxoid fibroma, Mayo Clinic experience. (From Dahlin DC: Bone Tumors: General Aspects and Data on 6,221 Cases. Third edition. Springfield, Illinois, Charles C Thomas, 1978, p 58. By permission.)

B). An osteoid osteoma located within the cancellous portion of the bone frequently induces less sclerotic reaction than does an osteoid osteoma located within the cortex. This lack of sclerosis is especially apparent if the lesion is located in an intracapsular location, such as the femoral neck (Fig. 9-21). The central portion of the nidus may show evidence of calcification. Sometimes this central calcification is the most prominent feature of an osteoid osteoma.*

A tumor in the end of the long bone may cause significant osteoporosis and also cause synovitis in the adjacent joint. In children, growth disturbances may be seen. In the spinal column, the lesion is usually found in the neural arch and almost invariably is located in the apex of the concave side of the curve (16).

If the routine roentgenogram is normal or equivocal and there is strong suspicion of osteoid osteoma, tomograms are very helpful (Fig. 9-20 *C*). These will also display the nidus when reactive sclerosis is extremely dense and obscures the lesion on the plain roentgenogram. Moreover, an osteoid osteoma will show intense uptake on bone scans. Scans are helpful in localizing the lesions (Fig. 9-20 *D*). Angiography also has been helpful in the diagnostic evaluation (17), showing a circumscribed blush in the early arterial phase.

The differential diagnosis includes conditions such as Brodie's abscess and chronic osteitis of Garré, and on rare occasions the new bone formation associated with an osteoid osteoma may simulate a primary malignant bone tumor. If the main

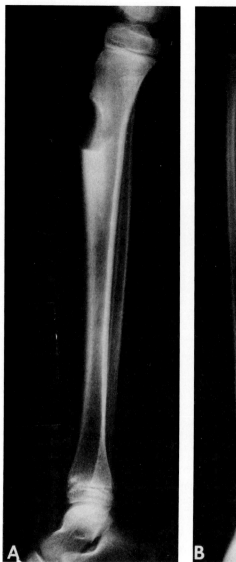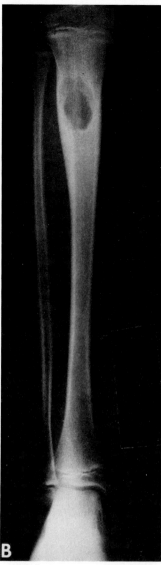

Fig. 9-14. Anteroposterior (*A*) and lateral (*B*) views of chondromyxoid fibroma of proximal tibia showing eccentric circumscribed area of rarefaction with a slightly scalloped margin.

finding is benign periosteal new bone formation, then a stress fracture also must be considered in the differential diagnosis.

Treatment is by surgical excision. The main problem with this type of surgery is the exact identification of the lesion, and for this reason, it is best done under roentgenographic control. A well-planned operative approach is essential. Proper identification of the nidus after en bloc removal is determined by roentgenograms and with the use of serial blocks by the pathologist (Fig. 9-20 *E*). Bone grafting may be required (Fig. 9-20 *F* and *G*).

If the lesion is not completely excised, the patient probably will continue to have pain and will require a second operation. Recently, we reviewed the records of 52 patients who had excision of a presumed osteoid osteoma, but no nidus was found (18). Twenty-nine of the patients had relief of their symptoms (22 after en bloc resection and 7 after curettage), but 23 had persistent symptoms. With persistence of typical symptoms of

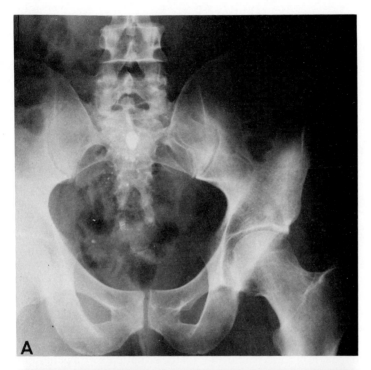

A

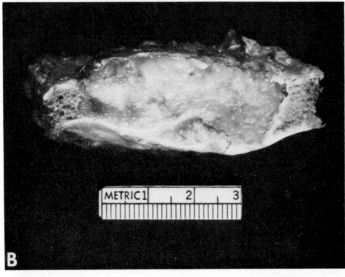

B

Fig. 9-15. *A*, Anteroposterior view of left ilium showing well-circumscribed area of rarefaction. The lesion was obscured by bowel gas and was missed on earlier roentgenograms. En bloc resection revealed chondromyxoid fibroma. *B*, Surgical specimen.

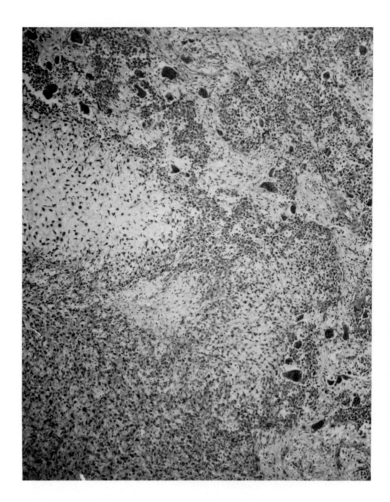

Fig. 9-16. Lobulated chondromyxoid fibroma with variable histologic features. Only rarely do these lesions have chondroid foci. (Hematoxylin and eosin: x64.)

an osteoid osteoma after surgery, one must have an aggressive attitude to treatment, and this demands complete reevaluation and reexploration, if indicated. Of the 23 patients with persistent symptoms, 18 had further surgery and 13 obtained relief. In 6 of these 13, no nidus was found at the second operation, but a nidus was confirmed in 7. Of the five patients with persistent symptoms after the second exploration, three had a third operation. All three patients obtained relief, and a nidus was discovered in two of the three. These interesting cases emphasize the importance of adequate resection of the lesion. In this group of patients, en bloc resection was performed in 50 patients and gave relief in 38, while curettage was performed in 22 and gave relief in 7. Curettage is to be discouraged because of the risk of leaving the nidus behind and of the difficulty in making a pathologic diagnosis of the specimen.

Osteoblastoma. Osteoblastoma, although histologically related to osteoid osteoma, is a progressively growing lesion of a larger size. The term "giant osteoid osteoma," synonymous with osteoblastoma, emphasizes the histologic similarity of this lesion

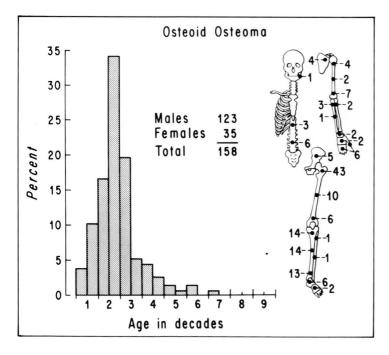

Fig. 9-17. Age and sex distribution of patients with osteoid osteoma, Mayo Clinic experience. (From Dahlin DC: Bone Tumors: General Aspects and Data on 6,221 Cases. Third edition. Springfield, Illinois, Charles C Thomas, 1978, p 76. By permission.)

to osteoid osteoma (14,19). Osteoblastomas have a predilection for the vertebral bodies and long bones. The 43 cases in the Mayo Clinic series (1) accounted for less than 1% of the primary tumors (Fig. 9-22). Approximately 70% were found in patients less than 20 years of age, with a pronounced predilection for males. While any bone may be involved, the bones of the vertebral column are commonly involved (Fig. 9-23). Patients with this tumor complain of a dull aching pain. Occurring insidiously, the lesion may be present for many months before the patient seeks medical attention. The pain pattern is not that commonly experienced with osteoid osteoma. Slight tenderness and palpable enlargement may be noted.

Scoliosis and muscle spasm occur in patients with spinal lesions. Neurologic deficits can be seen because of its frequent location near the spinal cord and emerging nerve roots. Another recently reported presentation is osteomalacia, which in two cases was noted to be cured by resection of the osteoblastoma (20).

Grossly, the tumor is larger than osteoid osteoma and is situated in cancellous bone. The tumor usually lacks the sclerotic reactive bone associated with osteoid osteoma. The tumor is fairly well circumscribed, red, granular, and friable. Older lesions may be much more heavily calcified, requiring decalcification before being cut.

Osteoblastomas present a variable microscopic appearance (Fig. 9-24). Some lesions show only slight osteoid formation with abundant fibrovascular connective tissue proliferation and

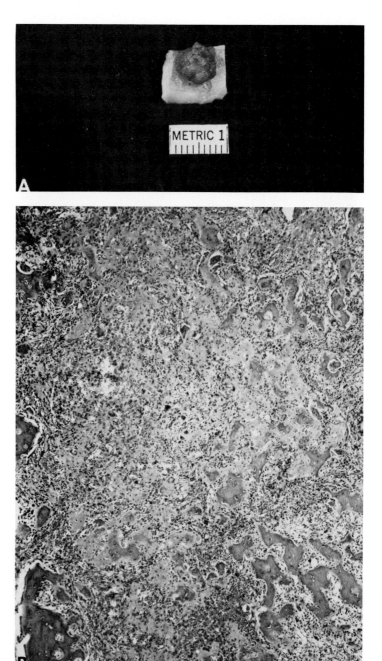

Fig. 9-18. *A*, Osteoid osteoma from distal femur of 15-year-old boy. Nidus is resting on a white sclerotic shell of bone. (From Dahlin DC: Bone Tumors: General Aspects and Data on 6,221 Cases. Third edition. Springfield, Illinois, Charles C Thomas, 1978, p 81. By permission.) *B*, Nidus of osteoid osteoma is composed of tightly woven thin trabeculae. Surrounding bone is frequently sclerotic. (Hematoxylin and eosin: x64.)

numerous giant cells, whereas other lesions show considerable osteoid formation. Mitotic figures may be found in the actively proliferating portion of the tumor. The osteoblasts, however, have abundant cytoplasm and lack nuclear atypia.

The roentgenographic appearance is quite varied and often not distinctive (18). However, the diagnosis can be suggested when the appearance is that of a large osteoid osteoma. Spinal lesions are usually expansile, and about half are mineralized.

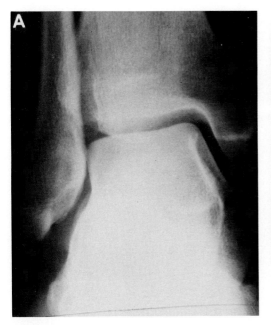 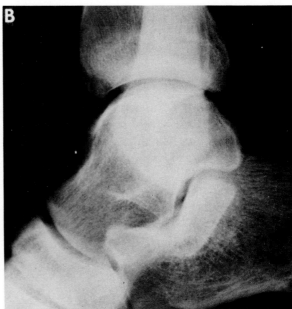

The benign nature of osteoblastoma dictates a conservative surgical approach, usually curettage (grade I) or excision (grade II). A wide margin of intact bone around the lesion is not required, and thorough curettage, cauterization, and bone grafting are usually successful. The major problem is with lesions involving the spinal column. In these instances, local excision is recommended, with preservation of the integrity of the spinal cord and emerging nerve roots. Surgical stabilization of the involved vertebral column may be indicated (Fig. 9-23). Radiation is contraindicated if the lesion is surgically accessible.

Fig. 9-19. *A* and *B*, Osteoid osteoma on anterior aspect of distal tibia showing typical lucent area. Patient had persistent pain for 2 years before discovery of lesion.

Tumors of Unknown Origin—Giant Cell Tumors

Giant cell tumor is a benign, locally aggressive lesion (21). The 264 cases in the Mayo Clinic series (22) accounted for 18.2% of the benign tumors (Fig. 9-25). It is one of the few bone tumors that is more common in females than males. Eighty-five percent of the neoplasms occurred in patients older than 20 years, with a peak incidence in the third decade of life. Patient age is helpful in differentiating the lesion from an aneurysmal bone cyst or a chondroblastoma, both of which occur in a younger age group. In the Mayo Clinic series, approximately half of the giant cell tumors were found in the distal femur and the proximal tibia. The lesions are found in the epiphyseal region of a long bone and extend up to the articular cartilage. When there are no physical signs or symptoms distinctly characteristic of giant cell tumor, the aggressiveness and the location of the tumor near

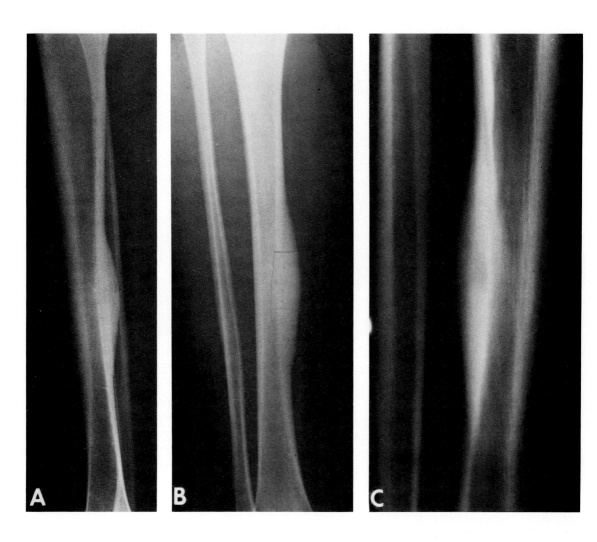

Fig. 9-20. Anteroposterior (A) and lateral (B) views of right tibia showing typical osteoid osteoma with lucent central nidus and surrounding active cortical sclerosis. C, Anteroposterior tomogram localizing the radiolucent nidus. D, Increased uptake is noted on radiographic bone scan. E, Lateral view of tibia after excision of lesion. Anteroposterior (F) and lateral (G) views of tibia demonstrating healing of bone grafts.

the joint usually result in intermittent aching pain, local swelling, tenderness, often limitation of motion, and a limp. A pathologic fracture may be the stimulus to seek medical attention, but usually the symptoms antedate the fracture. A tumor located in the spinal column or sacrum often presents with neurologic disturbances. The roentgenogram usually shows that the lesion is very destructive. The lesion may appear to be very aggressive, with a suspicion of malignancy. When a giant cell tumor is located at the end of a long bone, the roentgenographic diagnosis is relatively easy to make. The tumor is nearly always purely lytic and eccentrically located, extending to involve the subarticular portion of the bone (Fig. 9-26). Giant cell tumors may be well marginated, or they may fade more gradually into the adjacent normal bone. A rim of surrounding sclerosis is exceedingly rare, and if seen, another diagnosis is suggested.

Periosteal new bone in a giant cell tumor is extremely rare in the absence of a pathologic fracture. A large lesion may lose its eccentricity within the bone and grow to involve most of the

Fig. 9-20.

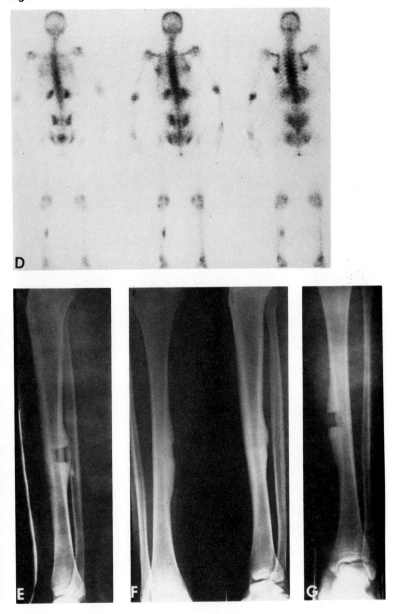

diameter and extend into the metaphyseal area. Commonly, trabeculations can be seen; these represent residual ridges of

Benign Tumors

cortex within the bone. A giant cell tumor may expand the cortex and may even destroy it, extending into the soft tissue. Pathologic fractures are not uncommon in aggressive-appearing lesions.

In tumors of the ilium and sacrum, the diagnosis is more difficult. Giant cell tumors tend to be subarticular in relation to the sacroiliac joint. Lesions in the spinal column are uncommon above the sacrum; when they do occur in the vertebral

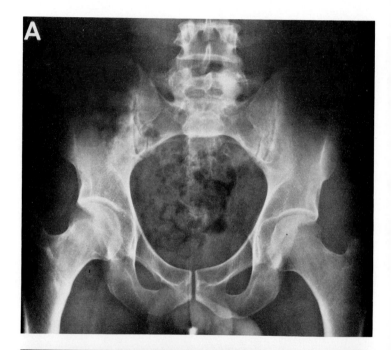

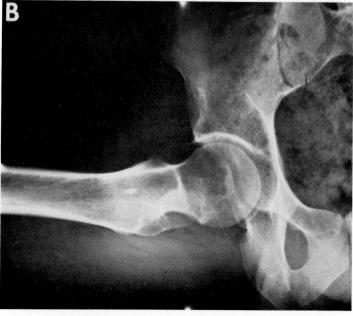

Fig. 9-21. Anteroposterior (A) and lateral (B) views of pelvis and femur. Patient had typical symptoms of osteoid osteoma in right hip, but lesion was difficult to detect. C and D, Tomographic views demonstrating nidus. E, Increased uptake localizing the nidus on bone scan.

134

Bone Tumors

column, they tend to be centered in the vertebral body, appearing as purely lytic lesions, and they may expand the bone. This is in contrast to aneurysmal bone cysts and osteoblastomas—lesions that are found more frequently in the posterior elements.

Postoperatively, when a giant cell tumor that has been grafted is evaluated, a recurrence is identified as an area of lucency at the graft site or of resorption of the bone grafts. Calcified de-

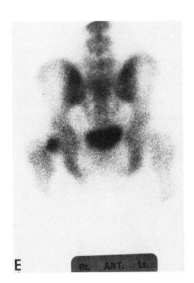

Fig. 9-21.

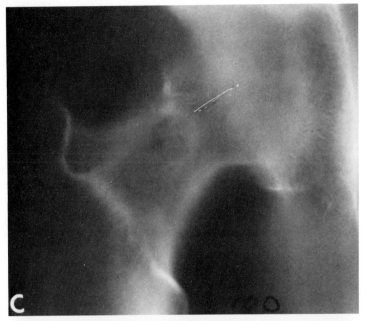

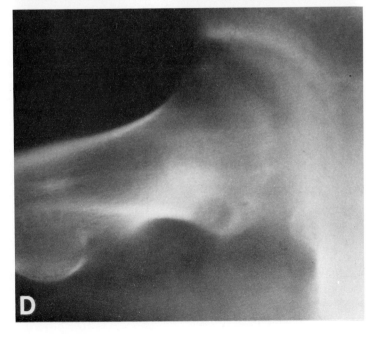

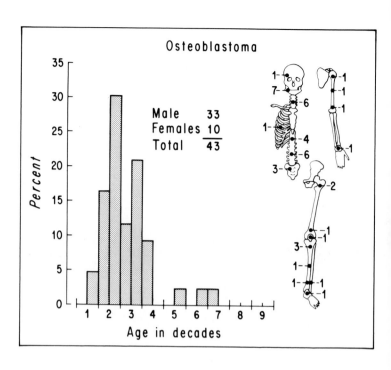

Fig. 9-22. Age and sex distribution of patients with osteoblastoma, Mayo Clinic experience. (From Dahlin DC: Bone Tumors: General Aspects and Data on 6,221 Cases. Third edition. Springfield, Illinois, Charles C Thomas, 1978, p 87. By permission.)

Table 9-1 Campanacci's Radiographic Classification of Giant Cell Tumor of Bone

Radiographic grade	Criteria
I	Quiescent, intraosseous
II	Active, periosteum intact
III	Aggressive, soft-tissue invasion

Modified from Merle d'Aubigné R, Thomine JM, Mazabraud A, et al: Évolution spontanée et post-opératoire des tumeurs à cellules géantes: indications thérapeutiques à propos de 39 cas dont 20 suivis 5 ans ou plus. Rev Chir Orthop 54:689–714, 1968

posits may be present within soft-tissue recurrences of a giant cell tumor. Campanacci and associates (23) have graded these lesions according to radiographic criteria (Table 1). This classification is helpful in selecting treatment. Grade I lesions are radiographically quiescent and appear to be relatively indolent. The lesions are small and entirely intraosseous. Grade II lesions appear to be more active. They have an aggressive roentgenographic appearance. These lesions may be more extensive, but the periosteum remains intact. Grade III lesions have a more aggressive appearance and extend beyond the periosteum and into the surrounding soft tissue.

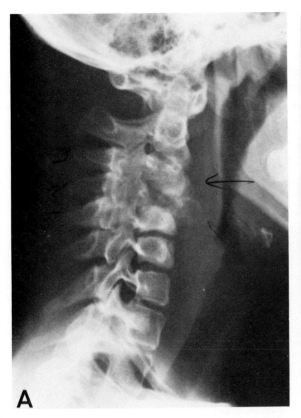 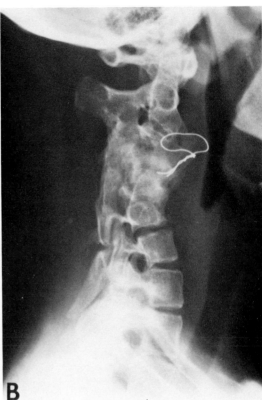

Grossly, the lesion is gray to red-brown and may show cystic change (Fig. 9-27 A). Yellow foci may be visible, owing to lipid-laden histiocytes. The tumor is characteristically soft and friable and nearly always extends to the articular surface.

Microscopically, the tumor is composed of proliferating round to oval mononuclear cells (Fig. 9-27 B). The mononuclear cells have an indistinct cytoplasm and are admixed with multinucleated giant cells. The nuclei of the giant cells are similar to nuclei of the mononuclear cells that surround them. Mitotic figures are present in practically every lesion; however, the nuclei of mononuclear cells and giant cells are not hyperchromatic or anaplastic. A giant cell tumor may have collagenic or even osteogenic foci, most commonly after fracture. The presence of chondroid foci, however, in a tumor with numerous giant cells should alert the pathologist that the lesion is not a benign giant cell tumor. In such cases, chondroblastoma is the most likely diagnosis, particularly if the chondroid foci are in islands. When there are zones of chondroid differentiation, one must also exclude the possibility of sarcoma.

Several cases have been reported in which the benign giant cell tumor has metastasized to the lungs (1). Although no patient has died of this condition, one patient in our experience had hundreds of small lesions in both lungs. In the lung, these met-

Fig. 9-23. *A,* Roentgenogram of cervical spinal column of 14-year-old girl showing destruction of C-4 due to osteoblastoma (*arrow*). This was associated with quadriparesis. *B,* After excision of lesion and anterior and posterior decompression with anterior cervical fusion of C-2 to C-5.

astatic lesions are seen histologically as a typical benign giant cell tumor that produces bone around the periphery, as there would be in soft-tissue recurrence.

We do not grade benign giant cell tumors histologically because there is no reliable grading system, nor has grading been helpful in predicting tumor behavior.

To be classified as a malignant giant cell tumor, the lesion must have areas of typical benign giant cell tumor mixed with areas of fibrosarcoma or osteosarcoma or must have a fibrosarcoma or an osteosarcoma at the site of a previously documented benign giant cell tumor that was treated with or without radiation. The presence of osteoclast-like giant cells in a malignant-appearing stroma is not adequate for the diagnosis of a malignant giant cell tumor. This definition, although arbitrary, has worked very well for us in relation to the clinical course of giant cell tumors. Included in the Mayo Clinic series of 264 patients were 20 patients with malignant giant cell tumor (1); in 13 of these 20, malignant giant cell tumors developed after radiation of benign giant cell tumors. Of the other seven patients, five had areas of sarcoma mixed with areas of benign giant cell tumor at the first operation, and two developed sar-

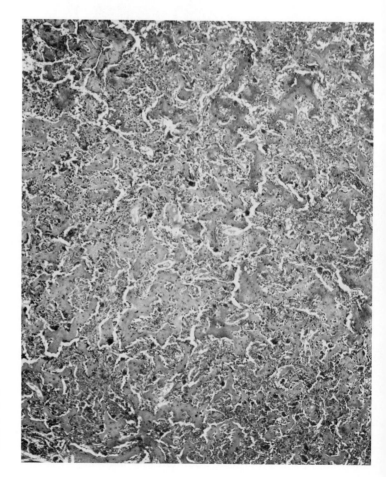

Fig. 9-24. Osteoblastomas have a variable histologic appearance. Considerable osteoid formation is present in lesion. Other tumors show less osteoid and more numerous giant cells. (Hematoxylin and eosin: x64.)

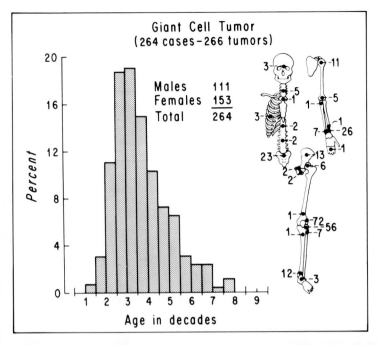

Fig. 9-25. Age and sex distribution of patients with giant cell tumor, Mayo Clinic experience. (From Dahlin DC: Bone Tumors: General Aspects and Data on 6,221 Cases. Third edition. Springfield, Illinois, Charles C Thomas, 1978, p 100. By permission.)

Fig. 9-26. *A*, Anteroposterior view of proximal tibia showing giant cell tumor. Lesion is eccentrically located and is thinning the cortex and extending to subarticular region. *B* and *C*, After wide exteriorization of lesion. Lesion has been curetted and cavity chemically cauterized with phenol and alcohol.

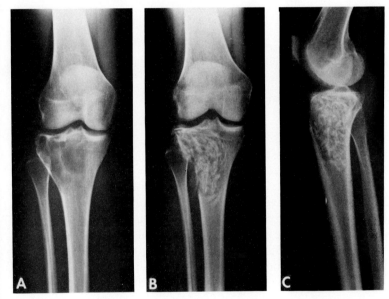

comas at sites of previously curetted benign giant cell tumors. This suggests that the giant cell tumor usually is a benign entity and should be treated as such, both initially and in recurrences.

The preoperative evaluation of giant cell tumors should include a routine medical evaluation to rule out such conditions as metastatic disease and the brown tumor of hyperparathy-

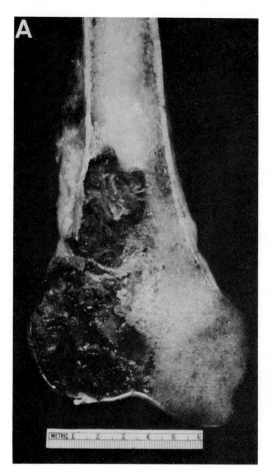

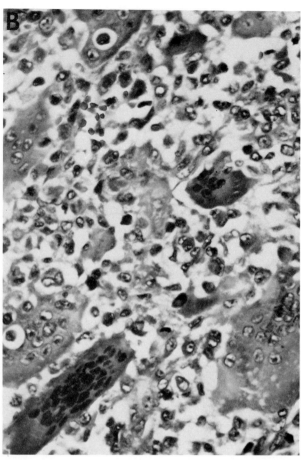

Fig. 9-27. *A,* Giant cell tumor is slightly atypical in its proximal extension in distal femur. Tumor extends to articular surface, as is characteristic of these lesions. *B,* Giant cell tumors are composed of admixture of mononuclear and multinucleated giant cells. Nuclei of these cells are morphologically similar and lack anaplasia and hyperchromatism. (Hematoxylin and eosin: x400.)

roidism. In order to assess the location of the tumor in relation to the popliteal vessels, in addition to routine roentgenograms, arteriograms have been helpful for evaluating knee lesions that have eroded the posterior cortex. Computed tomography is very useful when the lesion is in the sacrum or pelvis. Bone scans are not particularly helpful in assessing giant cell tumors.

In the treatment of this tumor, as of other lesions, careful preoperative planning and execution of the biopsy are extremely important, as outlined in Chapter 4. Because of the usual location of the giant cell tumor, the challenge is to remove all the tumor and preserve or restore the function of the neighboring joint. Although resection gives the best chance for cure, this necessitates sacrificing the joint, with severe alteration of function. A decision must be made regarding the extent of surgery necessary to balance the risk of recurrence against the functional deficit resulting from the surgery. The main factors to consider are the anatomic site of the lesion, the extent of the lesion, and the clinical and radiographic assessments of the aggressiveness of the tumor. In lesions in expendable bones, such as the fibula (Fig. 9-28), ulna, rib, and bones of the hand and foot, complete

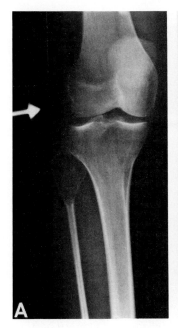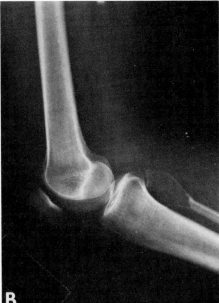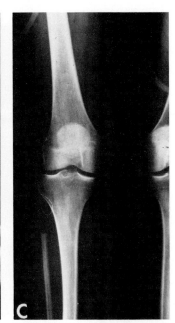

resection can be done without severe alteration in function. Unfortunately, about 50% of giant cell tumors are located in the region of the distal femur or upper tibia, and resection necessitates a major reconstruction effort in order to create an arthrodesis of the knee (Fig. 9-29) or to replace the excised bone with an allograft or a metallic implant (Fig. 9-30).

In our experience, curettage and grafting, used in an effort to preserve joint function, are associated with a recurrence rate of approximately 50%. However, for selected patients with lesions in long bones who were initially treated at our institution, this rate decreased to 25%.

As previously stated, the radiographic grading system of Campanacci and associates (23) is useful for planning surgery. The higher the radiographic grade, the more radical the surgery must be (Table 2). The tumor selected for curettage should be relatively small, radiographically quiescent, and entirely interosseous. The only significant risk encountered with curettage in these selected patients is that of recurrence. The risks of metastasis of residual or recurrent tumor and malignant transformation are essentially negligible and are not a consideration in determining the initial surgical procedure. If the initial lesion is large, has an aggressive appearance, and has broken through the cortex, a complete resection is indicated. The problem is that most tumors are in the middle zone between being small and entirely interosseous and being large with cortical destruction (Campanacci grade II). Such tumors require considerable judgment in planning treatment. Moreover, some patients are willing to accept the risk of recurrence if there is a reasonable

Fig. 9-28. Anteroposterior (*A*) and lateral (*B*) views of knee showing giant cell tumor involving proximal fibula. *C*, After resection.

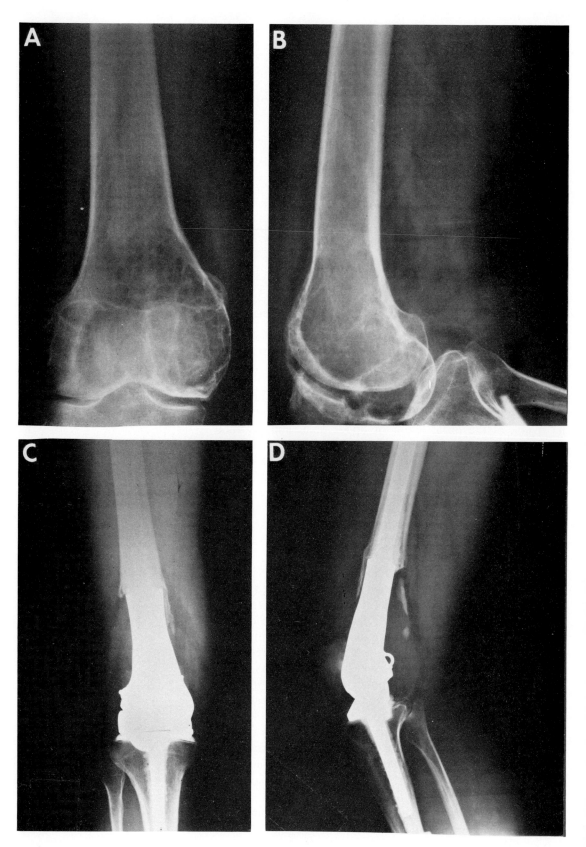

Table 9-2. Treatment Suggestions for Selected Anatomic Sites and Radiographic Grade

Anatomic site	Radiographic grade (Campanacci)		
	I	II	III
Distal femur or proximal tibia	Curettage and graft	Curettage or resection	Resection / arthrodesis or custom prosthesis
Proximal fibula	Resection	Resection	Resection
Distal radius	Curettage and graft	Curettage or resection	Resection / fibular autograft or arthrodesis

chance of avoiding sacrifice of a major joint, while others prefer to undergo a complete resection at the initial encounter despite the functional impairment. The measures that must be taken if curettage is to be successful have been outlined in Chapter 4. Critical to effective curettage and grafting is complete exteriorization of the lesion. Depending on the size of the lesion, excision-curettage may be effective (Fig. 9-31), but this is still a grade I surgical procedure. We utilize chemical cauterization with phenol and acid alcohol. More recently, others prefer to use methyl methacrylate.

Giant cell tumors not only can recur in bones and soft tissue but also can be transplanted to the bone graft donor site. Therefore, all bone grafts must be taken with a complete second surgical setup, including separate gloves, new instruments, and possibly repreparing and redraping the patient if there is a question of cross contamination. When resection is indicated, the entire end of the bone usually does not need to be removed, and when the tumor penetrates the surrounding soft tissues, the envelope of soft tissues must be removed in the resection. Reconstruction after the resection depends on the anatomic site, and these procedures are described in Chapter 8, on limb-salvage techniques. Amputation is indicated only for advanced lesions in which there is massive destruction of the bone near the major joint, especially after multiple recurrences or secondary infections. Radiation therapy is not recommended, except in the clinical situation in which the tumor cannot be excised. For example, a large giant cell tumor of the sacrum may not be resectable and may require radiation treatment.

Another situation that presents a therapeutic challenge is the presence of multicentric giant cell tumors, not only because the patient must be considered as a whole but also because each lesion must be assessed individually. While this condition is extremely rare, 7 cases of multicentric giant cell tumors have been documented in the literature, and 11 additional cases have

Fig. 9-29. Anteroposterior (A) and lateral (B) views of distal femur showing extensive recurrent giant cell tumor. Anteroposterior (C) and lateral (D) views of distal femur showing custom total knee arthroplasty.

been reported from the Mayo Clinic (20). In these conditions, treatment is influenced by the benign histologic characteristics of the tumor, and each patient is treated with local excision, curettage, or resection, depending on the circumstances.

Tumors of Fibrogenic Origin

Fibroma. Fibroma of bone (24-27) generally includes nonossifying or nonosteogenic fibroma, metaphyseal fibrous defect, fibrous cortical defect, and xanthofibroma. These fibrous lesions

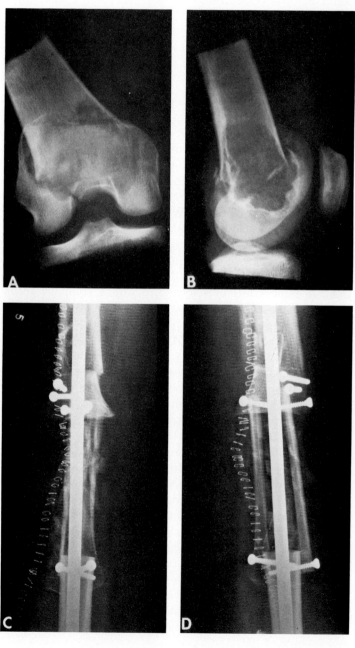

Fig. 9-30. *A* and *B*, Roentgenograms of resected specimen of distal femur. Patient has a Campanacci grade III giant cell tumor. Pathologic fracture is present. *C* and *D*, Surgical roentgenograms showing reconstruction of extremity with a segmental arthrodesis.

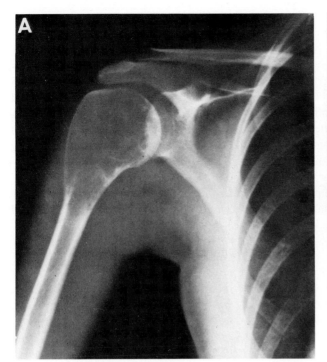
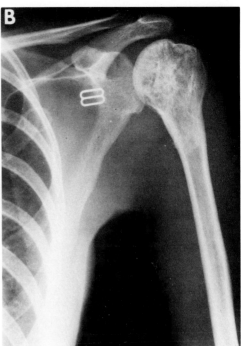

Fig. 9-31. *A,* Anteroposterior view of left proximal humerus showing extensive destruction from giant cell tumor. *B,* No evidence of recurrence 4¹/₂ years after radical exteriorization curettage and bone grafting.

probably represent a defect in ossification rather than neoplasm. The periosteal desmoid is another, less cellular, variant of these fibrous tumors (28,29). Trauma has been implicated in the pathogenesis. The fibrous cortical defect is a small, usually asymptomatic, intracortical lesion. Nonossifying fibroma is a larger lesion involving the medullary cavity of the bone. However, both are referred to as metaphyseal fibrous defects. The 72 fibromas in the Mayo Clinic series (1) constituted only 5% of the benign bone tumors, but the true incidence is probably much higher (Fig. 9-32). Fibroma in its classic form is almost exclusively a disease of childhood and adolescence and has been noted in 30 to 40% of all normal children older than 2 years. In the Mayo Clinic series, 85% of the patients were in the first two decades of life and males predominated. Although the patient is usually asymptomatic, and the lesion is found coincidentally, there may be slight swelling or localized pain if the lesion is large enough. Occasionally, the patient may present with a pathologic fracture, especially if he or she is an active adolescent.

Pathologically, the lesion is sharply demarcated from the surrounding bone and most often has several distinct lobules (Fig. 9-33). The tissue is usually red and granular but may have a yellow or brown foci if lipid or hemosiderin is present.

Microscopically, the lesion consists of spindle cells arranged in a storiform pattern. Foci of lipid-laden histiocytes are often noted. Hemosiderin pigment is frequently noted within the spindle cells. Mitotic figures are usually easily found in these lesions and should not dissuade the pathologist from making the diagnosis of this benign lesion.

Radiographically, the lesion is fairly characteristic and located eccentrically in the metaphyseal region of the bone, along with slight bulging of the cortical outline and a multiloculated appearance (Fig. 9-34). The lesion is usually very well marginated, often with a thin, smooth, scalloped rim of sclerosis around it. The long axis of the lesion is usually parallel with the long axis of the bone. Multiplicity of lesions is sometimes an important clue to diagnosis.

Treatment of the lesion depends on three factors: the certainty of the diagnosis, the structural integrity of the bone, and the proximity of the lesion to the epiphyseal plate. Clinically, with the characteristic roentgenographic appearance, most of these lesions do not require biopsy to confirm their nature. Generally, treatment is not necessary unless the lesion occupies more than 50% of the diameter of the bone or extends more than 3 or 4 cm into the bone. For lesions that pose a threat of a pathologic fracture, curettage and bone grafting are curative.

Desmoplastic Fibroma. Desmoplastic fibroma of bone as an entity has been well described in the recent literature (28,29). It is an extremely rare lesion that affects patients of all ages and is most commonly found in the metaphyseal region of long bones. Roentgenographically, the rarefying defect is generally central and reasonably well demarcated, often having an irreg-

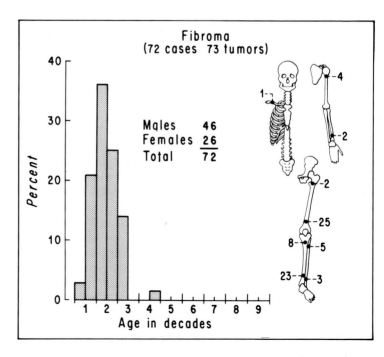

Fig. 9-32. Age and sex incidence of patients with fibroma, Mayo Clinic experience. (From Dahlin DC: Bone Tumors: General Aspects and Data on 6,221 Cases. Third edition. Springfield, Illinois, Charles C Thomas, 1978, p 123. By permission.)

ular border that produces a trabeculated appearance. Pain or swelling, sometimes of long duration, before the diagnosis is made is the commonest complaint and is accompanied by functional disability. A pathologic fracture occasionally may be the presenting symptom. Pathologically, the tumor can be considered the intraosseous counterpart of the desmoid tumor in the soft tissues. Grossly, the lesion is a dense, rubbery, firm, white mass of fibrous tissue. Microscopically, the tumor is hypocellular and composed of slender spindle-shaped cells with abundant collagen formation. Mitotic figures are absent or extremely rare. The nuclei are not atypical. Giant cells and osseous metaplasia are not features of this tumor.

Tumors of Vascular Origin—Hemangiomas

Hemangioma of bone is a benign vascular tumor. Sixty-nine lesions in the Mayo Clinic series (30) composed only 1.1% of

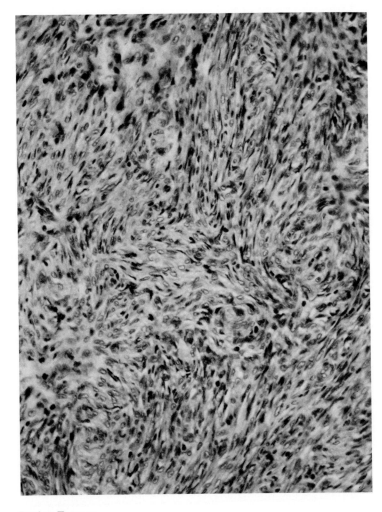

Fig. 9-33. Storiform pattern of metaphyseal fibrous defect. Hemosiderin pigment and lipid-laden histiocytes also are present. (Hematoxylin and eosin; x250.)

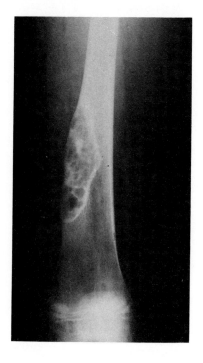

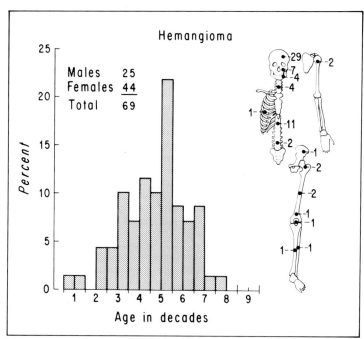

Fig. 9-34. Anteroposterior view of distal right femur showing nonossifying fibroma. There is a multiloculated appearance, with a thick rim of surrounding sclerosis. Lesion extends along long axis of femur.

Fig. 9-35. Age and sex incidence of patients with hemangioma, Mayo Clinic experience. (From Dahlin DC: Bone Tumors: General Aspects and Data on 6,221 Cases. Third edition. Springfield, Illinois, Charles C Thomas, 1978, p 138. By permission.)

the total series (Fig. 9-35). Nearly twice as many occurred in females, and one-third of the patients were in the fifth decade of life. Two-thirds of the hemangiomas occurred in the calvarium or vertebrae, and many of them affected the jaws (30).

Most hemangiomas of bone are solitary lesions; however, multiple bones in an extremity may be involved and may result in malformation of the extremity with dysfunction. Most hemangiomas are found in adults, and there is a predilection for the vertebral bodies and calvarium. "Disappearing" or "phantom" bone disease, also referred to as Gorham's disease (31), is also related to hemangioma-like proliferations in the bone. This rare condition more often affects children or young adults. Although the condition is self-limited, progression of this process is unpredictable.

The lesions are usually too widespread for effective surgical treatment, and radiation and chemotherapy do not appear to influence the already unpredictable course. The hemangiomas in the Mayo Clinic series (30), however, were usually asymptomatic and were discovered during roentgenographic study for other reasons. Local pain may be a feature, including compression fractures of the vertebrae. In most cases, the plain roentgenographic findings are characteristic. Lesions in the vertebrae cause rarefaction, with exaggerative vertical striations or a honeycombed appearance (Fig. 9-36). Calvarial lesions are lucent lesions with osseous spicules radiating from a central point, causing a typical "sunburst" appearance.

Grossly, these lesions are red to blue and may appear to be

honeycombed. If the tumor is firm without obvious vessels, the pathologist should carefully assess the tumor histologically, as it may be a malignant vascular tumor of bone. The histologic evaluation of vascular lesions of bone is difficult. On the obviously benign end of the spectrum, the lesions are characterized by widely dilated channels lined by flattened, inconspicuous endothelial cells or, less commonly, conglomerations of small vessels. In these cases, the pathologist must differentiate the hemangiomas from the hamartomatous malformations. More cellular lesions with plumper endothelial cells may be difficult to distinguish from low-grade sarcomas.

Hemangiomas usually respond well to conservative surgical procedure with curettage and grafting, but their infrequence and usually asymptomatic presentations usually make this unnecessary. The chief problems are encountered with the symp-

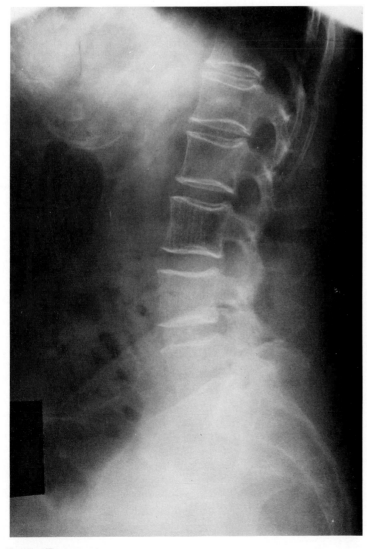

Fig. 9-36. Lateral view of lumbar spinal column showing typical hemangioma with exaggerated vertical striations.

tomatic spinal lesion. The higher morbidity and mortality rates that accompany surgical treatment are due to profuse hemorrhage. Because of these hazards, surgical treatment with laminectomy is reserved for patients with spinal cord compression. Spinal angiography is very helpful in these patients. Our preferred treatment in the symptomatic spinal lesion is radiation therapy with a dose of 3,000 or 4,000 rads.

References

1. Dahlin DC: Bone Tumors: General Aspects and Data on 6,221 Cases. Third edition. Springfield, Illinois, Charles C Thomas, 1978
2. Takigawa K: Chondroma of the bones of the hand: a review of 110 cases. J Bone Joint Surg [Am] 53:1591–1600, 1971
3. Rahimi A, Beabout JW, Ivins JC, et al: Chondromyxoid fibroma: a clinicopathologic study of 76 cases. Cancer 30:726–736, 1972
4. de Santos LA, Spjut HJ: Periosteal chondroma: a radiographic spectrum. Skeletal Radiol 6:15–20, 1981
5. Lichtenstein L, Hall JE: Periosteal chondroma: a distinctive benign cartilage tumor. J Bone Joint Surg [Am] 34:691–697, 1952
6. Lewis RJ, Ketcham AS: Maffucci's syndrome: functional and neoplastic significance; case report and review of the literature. J Bone Joint Surg [Am] 55:1465–1479, 1973
7. Ewing J: Cited by Huvos AG, Marcove RC, Erlandson RA, et al: Chondroblastoma of bone: a clinicopathologic and electron microscopic study. Cancer 29:760–771, 1972
8. Codman EA: Epiphyseal chondromatous giant cell tumors of the upper end of the humerus. Surg Gynecol Obstet 52:543–548, 1931
9. Jaffe HL, Lichtenstein L: Benign chondroblastoma of bone: a reinterpretation of the so-called calcifying or chondromatous giant cell tumor. Am J Pathol 18:969–991, 1942
10. Huvos AG, Marcove RC: Chondroblastoma of bone: a critical review. Clin Orthop 95:300–312, 1973
11. Dahlin DC, Ivins JC: Benign chondroblastoma: a study of 125 cases. Cancer 30:401–413, 1972
12. Schajowicz F, Gallardo H: Chondromyxoid fibroma (fibromyxoid chondroma) of bone: a clinicopathological study of thirty-two cases. J Bone Joint Surg [Br] 53:198–216, 1971
13. Jaffe HL: "Osteoid-osteoma": a benign osteoblastic tumor composed of osteoid and atypical bone. Arch Surg 31:709–728, 1935
14. Schajowicz F, Lemos C: Osteoid osteoma and osteoblastoma: closely related entities of osteoblastic derivation. Acta Orthop Scand 41:272–291, 1970
15. Sim FH, Dahlin DC, Stauffer RN, et al: Primary bone tumors simulating lumbar disc syndrome. Spine 2:65–74, 1977
16. Keim HA, Reina EG: Osteoid-osteoma as a cause of scoliosis. J Bone Joint Surg [Am] 57:159–163, 1975
17. O'Hara JP III, Tegtmeyer C, Sweet DE, et al: Angiography in the diagnosis of osteoid-osteoma of the hand. J Bone Joint Surg [Am] 57:163–166, 1975
18. Marsh BW, Bonfiglio M, Brady LP, et al: Benign osteoblastoma: range of manifestations. J Bone Joint Surg [Am] 57:1–9, 1975
19. McLeod RA, Dahlin DC, Beabout JW: The spectrum of osteoblastoma. Am J Roentgenol 126:321–335, 1976
20. Yoshikawa S, Nakamura T, Takagi M, et al: Benign osteoblastoma as a cause of osteomalacia: a report of two cases. J Bone Joint Surg [Br] 59:279–286, 1977
21. Larsson S-E, Lorentzon R, Boquist L: Giant-cell tumor of bone: a demographic, clinical, and histopathological study of all cases recorded

in the Swedish Cancer Registry for the years 1958 through 1968. J Bone Joint Surg [Am] 57:167–173, 1975

22. Dahlin DC, Cupps RE, Johnson EW Jr: Giant-cell tumor: a study of 195 cases. Cancer 25:1061–1070, 1970
23. Campanacci M, Giunti A, Olmi R: Giant-cell tumours of bone: a study of 209 cases with long-term follow-up in 130. Ital J Orthop Traumatol 1:249–277, 1975
24. Jaffe HL, Lichtenstein L: Non-osteogenic fibroma of bone. Am J Pathol 18:205–221, 1942
25. Hatcher CH: The pathogenesis of localized fibrous lesions in the metaphyses of long bones. Ann Surg 122:1016–1030, 1945
26. Ponseti IV, Friedman B: Evolution of metaphyseal fibrous defects. J Bone Joint Surg [Am] 31:582–585, 1949
27. Cunningham JB, Ackerman LV: Metaphyseal fibrous defects. J Bone Joint Surg [Am] 38:797–808, 1956
28. Kimmelstiel P, Rapp I: Cortical defect due to periosteal desmoids. Bull Hosp Joint Dis 12:286–297, 1951
29. Sugiura I: Desmoplastic fibroma: case report and review of the literature. J Bone Joint Surg [Am] 58:126–130, 1976
30. Unni KK, Ivins JC, Beabout JW, et al: Hemangioma, hemangiopericytoma and hemangioendothelioma (angiosarcoma) of bone. Cancer 27:1403–1414, 1971
31. Gorham LW, Stout AP: Massive osteolysis (acute spontaneous absorption of bone, phantom bone, disappearing bone): its relation to hemangiomatosis. J Bone Joint Surg [Am] 37:985–1004, 1955

CHAPTER 10

LESIONS SIMULATING TUMORS OF BONE

Thomas C. Shives, M.D.
Kay L. Cooper, M.D.
Lester E. Wold, M.D.

It is my impression that in the matter of recognizing and treating skeletal tumors in general more mischief is done currently through overdiagnosis than through failure to recognize malignant neoplasms promptly. *Lichtenstein*

Few surgeons realize the limitations in the histological diagnosis of bone tumors and the conditions which simulate or accompany them. *Ewing*

Although this book is devoted to skeletal tumors, it is important to recognize that certain conditions may simulate true neoplastic disease, benign or malignant. The mistaken identification of the underlying pathologic process may, on the one hand, merely result in delay of appropriate treatment, but on the other, it may result in the tragic amputation of a limb for benign disease. Therefore, the surgeon, radiologist, and pathologist must be cognizant of the reactive, traumatic, infectious, and other conditions of bone that may simulate neoplasia. Typical examples include osteomyelitis mistaken for Ewing's sarcoma, hyperparathyroidism misdiagnosed as giant cell tumor, and myositis ossificans misinterpreted as osteogenic sarcoma.

It is in the recognition of these "nontumors" that the interaction of surgeon, radiologist, and pathologist takes on immense proportions. This chapter is devoted to familiarizing the physician with the clinical, roentgenographic, and pathologic features of various lesions that may be easily mistaken for neoplasms. It is hoped that the physician may thereby avoid inappropriate biopsy and unwarranted therapy.

Unicameral Bone Cyst

The cause of solitary unicameral bone cyst is unknown, but according to Morton (1), the most plausible explanation is that it is due to an aberration of bone growth at the epiphyseal plate resulting from either trauma or hemorrhage. The condition is relatively common and manifests itself mainly in childhood and adolescence. It nearly always develops in the shaft of one of a few predilected long bones. In larger series (2–4), more than half of the cysts have been located in the upper part of the shaft of the humerus and in the proximal shaft of the femur. Other sites in long bones include the proximal and distal tibia, mid and distal humerus, distal femur, fibula, radius, and ulna (2–4). Nontubular bones are rarely affected.

Unicameral cysts are usually far advanced in their evolution before they are discovered. Generally, the cyst is detected only after a pathologic fracture has occurred. In a Mayo Clinic series (4), approximately half of the cysts were active (abutting an epiphysis) and half were latent (separated from the epiphysis by normal bone) at the time of first examination.

Because of the usual lack of physical findings preceding the pain secondary to spontaneous fracture, diagnosis before surgery is usually based on typical roentgenographic findings.

The unicameral bone cyst is seen roentgenographically as an elongated lucency centered within the medullary portion of the bone. Residual ridges of cortex may produce a trabeculated appearance (Fig. 10–1). With growth of the host bone, the cyst appears to migrate away from the epiphyseal plate. Unicameral bone cysts are usually widest at the epiphyseal end, but not wider than the epiphyseal plate. Periosteal new bone is absent unless a fracture has occurred. Although the roentgenographic findings are characteristic, a solitary bone cyst occasionally can produce an appearance closely resembling fibrous dysplasia, nonossifying fibroma, enchondroma, histiocytosis X, and even the early stages of osteogenic sarcoma.

Grossly, the cyst may contain a clear or yellow-green fluid.

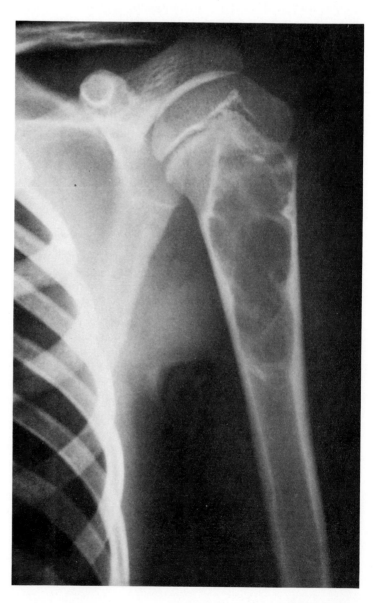

Fig. 10–1. Unicameral bone cyst centered within proximal humerus.

Bone Tumors

Some cysts are septated, and their gross appearance also may be altered by pathologic fracture. Histologically, the cyst is lined by a very thin layer of fibrous tissue. Thicker areas are composed of fibrous tissue with an admixture of benign giant cells and lymphocytes. The microscopic appearance also may be altered by pathologic fracture.

Therapeutic intervention, as opposed to watchful waiting, is usually indicated for all but small, resolving simple cysts in order to establish an accurate histologic diagnosis and prevent pathologic fracture, if it has not already occurred. Until recently, most authorities have agreed that surgical intervention is indicated and best done by thorough curettage and grafting of the defect with autogenous bone grafts (4, 5). However, Scaglietti et al. (6) reported in 1979 on 72 patients with unicameral cysts treated by topical injection of methylprednisolone acetate. All patients were followed up for 1 to 3 years, with favorable results in approximately 90% (that is, healing or enough bone repair to eliminate the risk of pathologic fracture). The authors emphasized the frequent need for repeat injections, especially in older patients (15 to 20 years of age).

As mentioned, unicameral bone cysts are distinctly rare in the nontubular bones. However, the literature contains reports of "solitary cysts" of the calcaneus. Cysts of the calcaneus deserve special attention because they are usually asymptomatic, detected incidentally, and when "typical," do not require treatment. The location of these cysts is constant. On the lateral roentgenographic view, the cyst is seen to occupy Ravelli's triangle, centered at the base of the neck just inferior to the anterior portion of the posterior facet. The lesion is triangular or oval and well-circumscribed. The diameters of the cysts vary from one-third to one-half the length of the calcaneus (7). On the tangential view, the cystic area is seen lying against the lateral cortex and involving one-half to two-thirds of the width of the bone (7, 8) (Fig. 10–2). When the above roentgenographic criteria are fulfilled, such lesions have been found to remain asymptomatic and stable in size, with no tendency for pathologic fracture. Although such lesions have been found to contain yellow fluid and possess a lining microscopically resembling that of the cysts seen in long bones, it is difficult to escape the impression that mechanical factors or a developmental abnormality may be responsible for the formation of these "cysts."

One should be suspicious of a cystic calcaneal lesion that differs from the lesions described above and should consider biopsy.

Aneurysmal Bone Cyst

Although an aneurysmal bone cyst may histologically resemble several other lesions of bone, it is now recognized as a separate and distinct entity (1). The lesion probably represents a reactive nonneoplastic process, similar to that seen with other

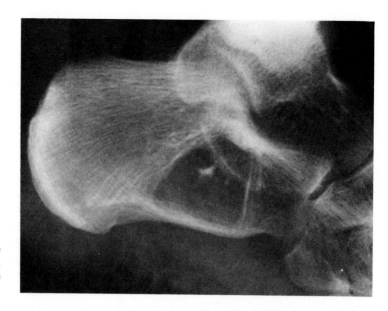

Fig. 10–2. Asymptomatic solitary bone "cyst" of calcaneus in 37-year-old man. (Roentgenogram courtesy of Dr. James Haemmerle, Menomonie, WI.)

reactive lesions of bone and periosteum or even heterotopic ossification. In diagnosing this lesion, one must be aware of two main pitfalls. First, aneurysmal bone cyst-like areas are found in various benign lesions, including unicameral bone cyst, giant cell tumor, chondroblastoma, chondromyxoid fibroma, and fibrous dysplasia (2). Second, aneurysmal bone cyst may be confused with telangiectatic osteosarcoma, because both their rapid growth patterns and histologic appearances may be similar. Failure to make this distinction may obviously result in serious therapeutic mismanagement.

The lesion may be seen in the vertebral column (usually posterior elements) or in flat or long bones. In Dahlin's collected series of 134 patients (2), 78% were less than 20 years old. By contrast, more than 80% of patients with giant cell tumor are 20 years old or older (2). Lesions of long bone are usually metaphyseal (again in contrast to giant cell tumor), although extension to the end of the bone may be seen after closure of the physis. Pain and swelling of variable duration are the usual presenting symptoms. With vertebral involvement, signs and symptoms may be secondary to compression of the cord or root.

Individual lesions are purely lytic and almost invariably expansile. Aneurysmal bone cysts most often are well circumscribed but lack a sclerotic border. Eccentric lesions, causing bulging and pronounced thinning of the overlying cortex, are most common (Fig. 10–3). Extremely rapid growth is characteristic and often apparent on serial films.

Microscopically, aneurysmal bone cyst-like areas may be found in various bone lesions, most of which are benign, although rarely such foci may be seen in malignant tumors. Because of this, a lesion should be designated aneurysmal bone cyst only if the entire specimen has that histologic pattern. Aneurysmal

Bone Tumors

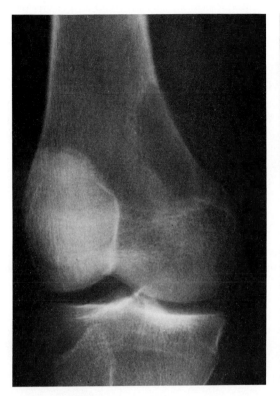 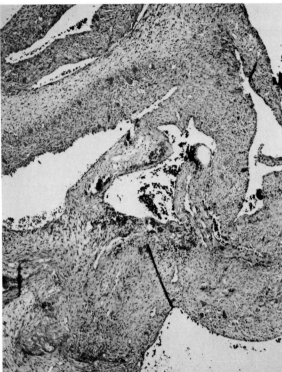

bone cysts are composed of cavernous spaces that lack an endothelial lining. The walls of the spaces are composed of fibrous tissue with an admixture of thin strands of "fiber-bone" (Fig. 10–4).

Treatment by curettage and grafting has generally been successful, although recurrence can be expected in 20 to 30% of cases (1). Wide exteriorization, allowing easy access to the entire lesion, is essential when this therapeutic modality is employed. For lesions in an expendable bone (for example, fibula or rib), en bloc resection is preferred. Although there are reports in the literature of favorable responses to treatment by radiation (3), three postradiation sarcomas in Dahlin's series have made us question its use.

Cysts Associated With Diseases of Joints

Cystic lesions of bone related to primary synovial disease may become large and produce a roentgenographic pattern that is suggestive of neoplasia.

Subchondral granulomatous lesions that are seen as cystic or

Fig. 10–3. Eccentric aneurysmal bone cyst in distal femoral metaphysis, expanding into adjacent soft tissues.

Fig. 10–4. Cystic spaces in aneurysmal bone cysts lack an endothelial lining. Benign proliferating fibroblasts, giant cells, and "fiber-bone" form the septae. (Hematoxylin and eosin; x64.)

lytic areas on the roentgenogram are frequent findings in rheumatoid arthritis. Similar lesions also occur in gout and degenerative arthritis and may be present in Charcot's joints, syphilitic arthritis, and hemophilic arthritis (1). In rheumatoid arthritis, subchondral cyst-like lesions commonly occur in the hands, wrists, and feet, but they may develop adjacent to major joints or in the vertebrae. The lesions may be seen at all stages of arthritic involvement, along with typical joint changes, but they also may be found without other roentgenographic evidence of rheumatoid disease.

Pigmented villonodular synovitis can involve soft tissues and bone extensively, especially about the hip and knee. Erosion of bone or formation of small, well-defined unilocular or multilocular cysts by the proliferating masses of synovial tissue may be mistaken for primary disease of bone (Fig. 10–5).

Occasionally, certain infectious processes such as tuberculosis or brucellosis involving joints may invade and destroy juxta-articular bone (2).

Ganglion Cysts of Bone

Intraosseous ganglia are rare, but they must be considered in the differential diagnosis when one is confronted with a sol-

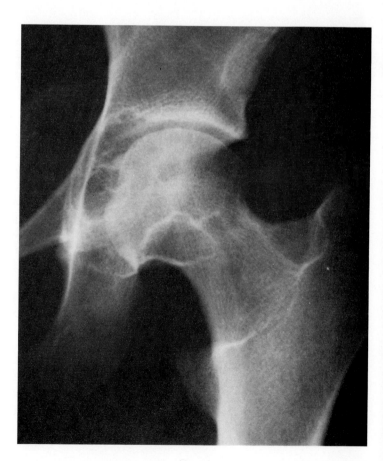

Fig. 10–5. Pigmented villonodular synovitis of hip, with erosive changes in both the femoral neck and acetabulum.

Bone Tumors

itary cyst of bone. These ganglia are most commonly seen in middle-aged adults, very near an adjacent joint. There is a predilection for bones about the ankle, especially the distal tibia. Other sites, in decreasing order of frequency, are the ulna, carpal bones, proximal femur, proximal tibia, acetabulum, distal femur, and tarsal bones (1). Symptoms, when present, usually consist of mild, intermittent, dull-aching discomfort about the joint, related to activity. Slight local swelling may be present (2).

The cause of these lesions remains unsettled. They may develop by the intrusion of an overlying soft-parts ganglion into bone (2), but in most cases, contiguity between intraosseous ganglia and soft-tissue components has not been demonstrated. Most authors believe that intraosseous ganglia arise de novo within bone. Feldman and Johnston (3) suggest that ganglia of bone result from a primary intramedullary fibroplasia, followed by a secondary cystic and degenerative stage.

Intraosseous ganglia are seen roentgenographically as a purely lytic lesion, usually in the epiphyseal end of a tubular bone. Their sizes vary from 2 mm to 7 cm (3). Sharp demarcation from the surrounding bone is evidence of their benign nature. Occasionally, marginal sclerosis and multiloculation are seen. No matrix mineralization is present. Periosteal new bone is also lacking, unless a pathologic fracture has occurred. Lesions in the end of a tubular bone are usually eccentric and have a subchondral location (Fig. 10–6). In the absence of secondary degenerative arthritis, the adjacent joint is normal. If the cyst is epiphyseal in location, differentiation from benign chondroblastoma and giant cell tumor may be difficult. Rarely, the lesion will present with a very aggressive, destructive appearance that will be suggestive of a malignant condition.

In our experience, intraosseous ganglion cysts may be most easily confused pathologically with the juxta-articular cysts of degenerative joint disease (Fig. 10–7).

Treatment by curettage and bone grafting is usually indicated. Recurrence after surgery is rare.

Pseudocysts of Humerus

Brief mention should be made of the frequently deceiving roentgenographic appearance of a rarefaction in the lateral portion of the humeral head. When pronounced, this rarefaction can be confused with a lytic neoplasm. Most of our referred cases have had a provisional diagnosis of giant cell tumor. Helms (1) evaluated 50 roentgenograms of the shoulder using projections made in internal and external rotation and found that only 2% had no rarefaction of the humeral head. Five patients (10%) had rarefaction that was so well defined that it could be easily confused with a lytic lesion (Fig. 10–8). The roentgenographic appearance is believed to be due to a lesser amount of trabecular bone in the greater tuberosity than in the remainder of the

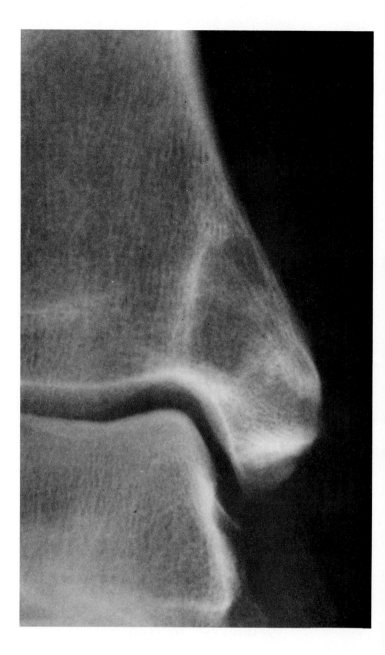

Fig. 10–6. Intraosseous ganglion in medial malleolus of 56-year-old man.

humeral head. The characteristic size and location, absence of cortical destruction, clear margins, and lack of periosteal reaction usually allow differentiation from more serious pathologic conditions. The typical finding is usually, but not always, bilateral. When doubt exists, follow-up films are recommended.

Recognition of this finding will avoid unnecessary biopsy.

Osteomyelitis

Inflammatory lesions may occasionally mimic neoplasms of bone, both clinically and roentgenographically. Failure to make

Bone Tumors

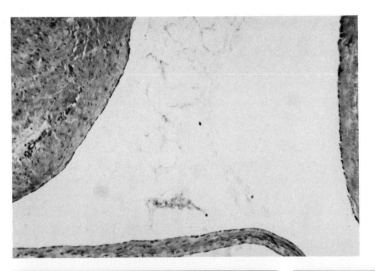

Fig. 10–7. Ganglion cysts rarely occur in bone. Typically, they are composed of thick fibrous wall and contain mucoid fluid. Histologically similar lesions can be seen associated with degenerative joint disease. (Hematoxylin and eosin; x350.)

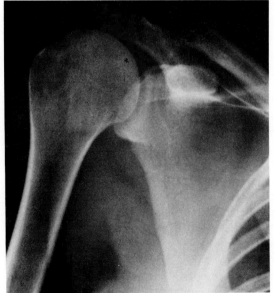

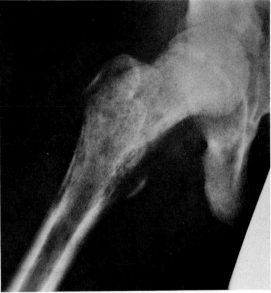

a correct differentiation may result in a delay of appropriate treatment when in fact there is a malignancy or may eventuate in unnecessary amputation as a result of "overdiagnosis" (1).

Osteomyelitis may mimic almost any tumor, although Ewing's sarcoma is the most commonly suspected neoplasm. At the Mayo Clinic, in a group of cases of proved osteomyelitis simulating neoplasia, suspected erroneous roentgenographic diagnoses included Ewing's sarcoma, reticulum cell sarcoma, leu-

Fig. 10–8. "Pseudocyst" of right humeral head in 23-year-old girl referred with provisional diagnosis of giant cell tumor.

Fig. 10–9. Acute osteomyelitis of proximal femur. Permeative pattern of destruction suggests malignant tumor, such as Ewing's sarcoma.

kemia, osteoid osteoma, benign cyst, chondromyxoid fibroma, and osteogenic sarcoma (2).

Usually, *acute* hematogenous osteomyelitis can be correctly diagnosed when the roentgenographic findings are considered in conjunction with a complete clinical history. The usual fever and sepsis of acute infection may, however, be obscured by antibiotic therapy. Also, Ewing's sarcoma can be accompanied by fever and leukocytosis.

When the patient has *subacute* or *chronic* osteomyelitis, the diagnosis can be difficult. Historical or laboratory evidence suggesting infection may be lacking, and the roentgenographic findings may be confusing, especially when they are altered by inadequate treatment.

The first roentgenographic sign of osteomyelitis is deep soft-tissue swelling, causing obliteration of the muscle planes. This swelling can be seen as early as 24 hours after the onset of symptoms. At this stage of the disease, isotope bone scans usually give positive findings, and this can be used to confirm the diagnosis. Destructive skeletal lesions and periosteal new bone formation become evident 7 to 12 days after the onset of symptoms. The irregular destruction in osteomyelitis is usually located in the metaphysis. Poorly marginated and permeative patterns of bone destruction are common and may be suggestive of a malignant process (Fig. 10–9). The periosteal reaction generally has a solid, benign appearance, although Codman's triangles may be seen in association with cortical destruction. Sequestra appear as dense separate fragments of bone within the destruction. The presence of lucent serpiginous tracks within the bone is another helpful sign of osteomyelitis. These roentgenographic features may become more apparent with conventional tomography. Septic arthritis and pathologic fractures may complicate acute osteomyelitis.

Subacute osteomyelitis usually appears as a more sharply marginated, less aggressive process. A rim of sclerosis often surrounds the lesion. In chronic osteomyelitis, the long-standing process produces cortical thickening and sclerosis. Lymphoma of bone must often be considered in the differential diagnosis. The recognition of sequestra and lucent tracks in these cases allows the diagnosis of osteomyelitis.

Although acute and chronic infections may produce roentgenographic changes that simulate those of bone tumors, histologically the differentiation of osteomyelitis from neoplasm is usually not difficult (2). Occasionally, subacute osteomyelitis may appear to be similar to histiocytosis X microscopically. On other occasions, an almost purely plasmacytic infiltrate will resemble myeloma (Fig. 10–10).

Treatment of presumed osteomyelitis should never be instituted without an adequate biopsy. A specimen for histologic examination should include an adequate amount of periosteum, cortical bone, and medullary tissue. A needle biopsy, despite its simplicity and advantage of reduced surgical trauma, may

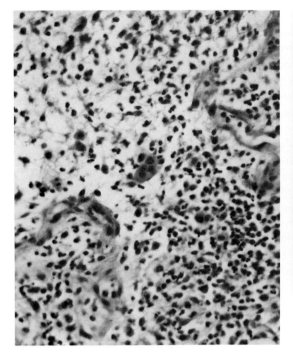

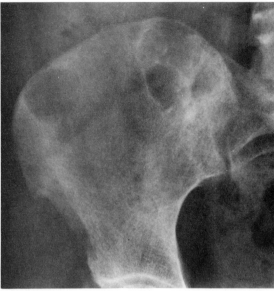

not provide a specimen representative of the lesion and thus may result in a delayed or erroneous diagnosis.

Therapeutic management of osteomyelitis varies with the organism responsible for the infection, including a wide variety of bacterial and mycotic agents. *Staphylococcus aureus* remains the most common offending organism.

In patients with long-standing chronic osteomyelitis, a draining sinus may develop. These patients are at risk of developing a superimposed squamous cell carcinoma. Suspicion should be aroused by exacerbation of chronic symptoms or a flare-up in the quiescent stage of infection (3).

Fig. 10–10. Histologically, osteomyelitis is characterized by mixture of polymorphonuclear leukocytes, lymphocytes, histiocytes, and plasma cells in varying numbers. (Hematoxylin and eosin; x400.)

Fig. 10–11. Brown tumors of ilium.

Hyperparathyroidism

The incidence of bone lesions in hyperparathyroidism varies from 30 to 40% (1). In advanced hyperparathyroidism, rarely seen in this era of early chemical diagnosis and swift surgical exploration, the entire skeleton may be involved. Pronounced local absorption sometimes produces an appearance of a cyst-like lesion on the roentgenogram (so-called brown tumor), which can simulate the appearance of a primary neoplasm (Fig. 10–11).

Occasionally, localized defects of parathyroid osteopathy produce a lesion similar to a giant cell tumor or even an aneurysmal bone cyst. Suspicion should be aroused when the findings are suggestive of the diagnosis of giant cell tumor but the histologic appearance or the skeletal location of the lesion is unusual or incorrect for giant cell tumor (2).

With more widespread skeletal changes of hyperparathyroidism, one may be led to suspect carcinomatosis or multiple myeloma or even senile or idiopathic osteoporosis (3). However, if one is aware of the possibility of hyperparathyroidism, confirmatory evidence of the diagnosis usually can readily be furnished by such findings as subperiosteal resorption of bone, mottling of the calvarium, nephrocalcinosis, and significant, well-known chemical alterations in the serum.

The histologic appearance in parathyroid osteopathy is not specific. Multiple bony lesions may be associated with hyperparathyroidism and are a clue to the correct diagnosis. The "brown tumor" of hyperparathyroidism is the end-stage result of the long-standing elevation of the parathyroid serum hormone level. These nodules are composed of multinucleated osteoclastic giant cells embedded in a loose fibrous stroma (Fig. 10–12). Histologically, the lesion may resemble giant cell tumor of bone; however, the fibrous nature of the lesion or the finding of an atypical location should alert the pathologist to the correct diagnosis. The "early" histologic changes of hyperparathyroidism may be seen in areas adjacent to a "brown tumor." These changes consist of osteoclastic tunneling through bony trabeculae and fibrosis of the surrounding marrow.

Paget's Disease of Bone

In the early stages of Paget's disease, resorptive changes are prominent and the resulting circumscribed defects may simulate a primary tumor of bone. These early lesions in the skull are recognized well enough to have been labeled "osteoporosis circumscripta cranii," but not so well appreciated is the fact that they may be seen in the pelvis, femur, tibia, and vertebrae,

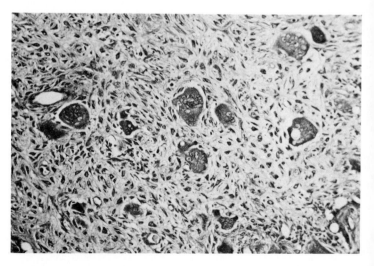

Fig. 10–12. Histologically, lesion of parathyroid osteopathy resembles benign giant cell tumor of bone. However, background stroma is more fibrogenic and spindled than in true giant cell tumor. (Hematoxylin and eosin; x600.)

Bone Tumors

occasionally causing confusion for both the surgeon and the radiologist (1). Paget's disease almost invariably extends to the end of a long bone. In the lytic phase, an appearance similar to a sharp blade of grass demarcates the area of involvement from the adjacent normal bone (Fig. 10–13). Characteristically, involved bones show enlargement, cortical thickening, and a coarse trabecular pattern (Fig. 10–14). Incomplete cortical fractures are common. Softening of bones produces basilar invagination, bowing of long bones, and acetabular protrusion.

With more widespread skeletal involvement by Paget's disease, differentiation from osteoblastic metastasis may be difficult. Widening or expansion of the involved bone, however, is reliable evidence that the sclerosing lesion is a manifestation of Paget's disease and not metastatic disease (2).

Paget's disease progresses through a number of stages. In the early stages, the histologic features are not specific and may resemble those of early lesions of hyperparathyroidism. Even in the later stages, roentgenologic bias is helpful in making the diagnosis of Paget's disease. In the late stages, the bony trabeculae are broad and irregular, with numerous reversal or "cement" lines (Fig. 10–15). The marrow surrounding these broad trabeculae shows a proliferation of bland fibrovascular connective tissue. These histologic features are not pathognomonic of Paget's disease, as similar bony changes may be seen in reactive and inflammatory conditions.

Treatment in early Paget's disease is symptomatic. If the disease remains localized, it is unlikely to have untoward consequences.

Avulsive Cortical Irregularity

Cortical irregularities of the distal femur in children and adolescents are frequent and may be mistaken for an inflammatory

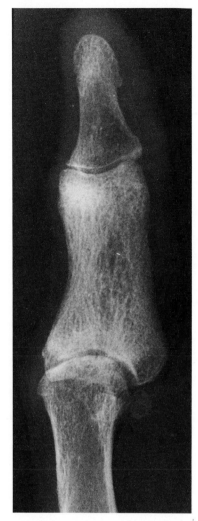

Fig. 10–14. Sclerosis and expansion of proximal phalanx of thumb due to Paget's disease.

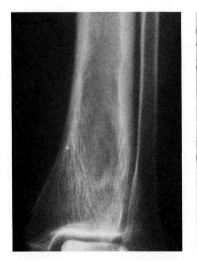 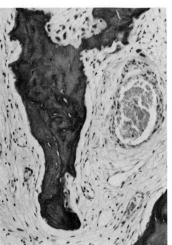

Fig. 10–13. Lytic phase of Paget's disease involving distal tibia. Blade-of-grass appearance is seen at proximal extent of lesion.

Fig. 10–15. Paget's disease is characterized by irregular broad trabeculae with numerous reversal or "cement" lines, as can be seen in this lesion involving the maxilla. Marrow is replaced by fibrovascular connective tissue. (Hematoxylin and eosin; x350.)

or malignant process. Because of suspected malignancy (1), many children have biopsy specimens taken. First described by Kimmelstiel and Rapp (2) in 1951, this abnormality has been variously referred to as periosteal desmoid, subperiosteal desmoid, subperiosteal abrasion, cortical abrasion, medial distal metaphyseal femoral irregularity, and subperiosteal cortical defect. Avulsive cortical irregularity seems to be the most appropriate term for this lesion because the presumed pathogenesis, general location, and roentgenographic appearance are implied by the name (3).

Usually, these lesions are quiescent and are not the cause of the symptoms for which a roentgenogram is taken. Avulsive cortical irregularity is most commonly seen in children who are 10 to 15 years old, but it has been found in children between 3 and 17 years of age. In a retrospective study of 345 knees in children, Simon (4) noted that the lesion was slightly more than three times as common in boys as in girls and approximately twice as common on the left than on the right side. The irregularity occurred in 11.5% of the males and 3.6% of the females studied (4). Young and co-workers (5), in a review of 350 roentgenograms of the knee, likewise found a male predominance but an equal incidence between the right and the left femur. The lesions are present bilaterally in approximately 35% of patients (3). The irregularities do not always disappear completely, but they decrease significantly in size at the time of epiphyseal closure (5).

The avulsive cortical irregularity has a very characteristic location, along the posteromedial aspect of the distal femoral metaphysis. Barnes and Gwinn (1) have performed dissection studies in this region and concluded that the irregularity is a normal finding and is due to the medial supracondylar ridge (the medial extension of the linea aspera). This ridge is formed owing to the aponeurosis of the extensor portion of the adductor magnus muscle and the associated muscle stress. In addition to the strong muscle pull exerted in this area, intense bone remodeling occurs simultaneously during periods of rapid skeletal growth. Presumably, during growth and remodeling, a disparity may develop between resorption and formation of cortical bone. Accelerated cortical bone resorption may result from the strong pull of the adductor muscle. This excessive mechanical stress may produce microavulsions of the cortical bone, eliciting a hypervascular and fibroblastic response, which in turn stimulates added osteoblastic activity and bone resorption (3).

In contrast to the normal, sharp cortical line proximal to the adductor tubercle, this lesion appears as a shallow, concave, irregular osteolytic lesion near the epiphysis, best seen with the knee externally rotated from 20 to 45°. The area of involvement is usually from 1 to 3 cm in length. Perpendicular bone spiculation may be present in the early phases. In the lateral projection, the lesion is seen as an area of cortical thickening. It may be irregular and, early during the course, may show a lamellated periosteal reaction with irregular ossification that resembles osteosarcoma (Fig. 10–16) (6).

There is no associated soft-tissue mass, and the adjacent soft-tissue planes are preserved. These roentgenographic features, combined with an absence of increased warmth, palpable mass, or tenderness on physical examination, should make the correct diagnosis apparent.

Occasionally, when some doubt exists regarding the roentgenographic findings, we obtain distal femoral tomograms with the patient's knee externally rotated. This allows the lesion to be precisely localized and confirms the absence of a soft-tissue mass.

Histologically, these lesions are composed of a loose admixture of hypocellular fibrous tissue that contains occasional be-

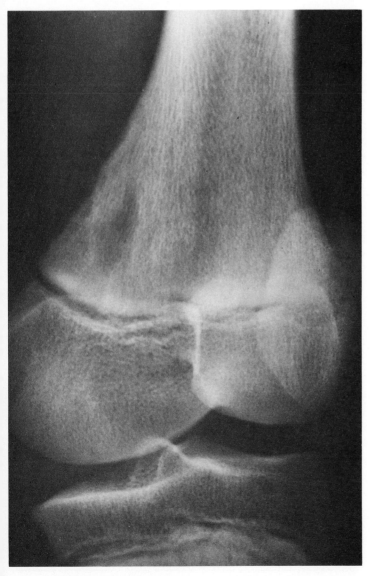

Fig. 10–16. Avulsive cortical irregularity on posterior medial aspect of distal femoral metaphysis.

Lesions Simulating Tumors of Bone

nign giant cells. The underlying cortical bone may be somewhat irregular. The characteristic location and bland histologic appearance are helpful in identifying this nonneoplastic process.

The ability to recognize this lesion on the roentgenogram allows differentiation from a malignant neoplasm, thus avoiding unnecessary biopsy.

Bone Infarcts

Bone infarcts are relatively common in people who work in compressed air (caisson workers) and in patients with sickle-cell anemia. However, skeletal lesions identical to those of caisson disease occur in persons not subject to air-pressure abnormalities, many of whom have had no symptoms. Bullough and others (1) have drawn attention to single and multiple bone infarcts of unknown cause occurring in various bones, other than the femoral head. These infarcts may be mistaken for calcifying cartilaginous neoplasms, cysts, and even osteoid osteoma with a surrounding halo of sclerotic bone (2).

These lesions, which generally are found in middle- to older-aged adults, involve most commonly the proximal tibia, distal femur, ilium, calcaneus, rib, distal tibia, fibula, and humerus (1). Usually metaphyseal when in a long bone, the lesions may be symmetrical. In approximately half of the patients in Bullough's series, the complaint (usually intermittent, dull-aching pain) could be reasonably attributed to the lesion seen on the roentgenogram. The pathogenesis in most cases is not clear. Previous authors have cited atherosclerosis, systemic immobilization, and local trauma as possible etiologic factors.

In the early stages of the disease, there may be no roentgenographic findings. Later, the findings consist of a region of rarefaction as the result of ischemic necrosis of cancellous bone. Gradually, areas of irregular density are seen as the result of ingrowth of new bone and impregnation of the necrotic zone with calcium salts. When fully developed, the disease has the typical appearance of a moderately thick serpentine border frequently outlining an elongated area of central lucency (Fig. 10–17). Despite the generally radiolucent center, irregular flecks of calcification consequent to fat necrosis are usually visible. The appearance may be likened to a coil of smoke (1). If the lesion is solitary, the appearance is most likely to be confused with that of a calcified enchondroma. In the latter lesion, however, the calcification is usually fairly uniform throughout, and its margins are not outlined so clearly.

Histologically, bone infarcts are characterized by necrotic osseous trabeculae and amorphous calcification of the intervening degenerated marrow (Fig. 10–18). None of the reactive cellular infiltrate associated with a bone infarct shows cytologic features of malignancy. Rarely, a sarcoma of bone (fibrosarcoma or osteosarcoma) may arise at the site of a bone infarct (3).

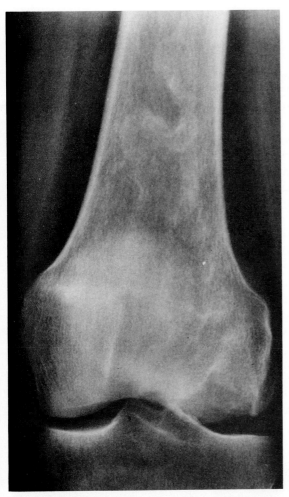 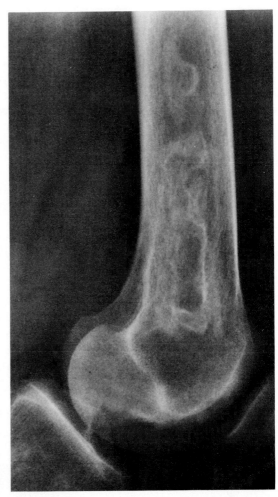

Fig. 10–17

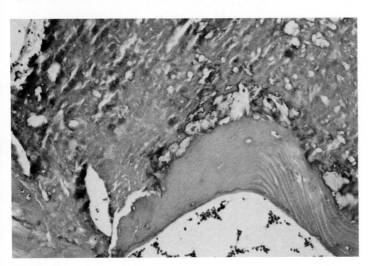

Fig. 10–18

Fig. 10–17. Anteroposterior (*A*) and lateral (*B*) views showing irregular sclerosis in distal femoral metaphysis due to bone infarction. Ischemia also has produced a large area of osteonecrosis in lateral femoral condyle.

Fig. 10–18. Bone infarcts are radiodense from mineralization of degenerated bone and marrow. Amorphous necrotic tissue is seen adjacent to residual normal bony trabeculae. (Hematoxylin and eosin; x540.)

Lesions Simulating Tumors of Bone

Bone Islands

Bone islands are benign, asymptomatic, osteosclerotic foci of trabecular bone frequently seen on the roentgenogram. Roentgenographically, bone islands are characterized by a small round or oval area of sclerosis with radiating spicules of thickened trabeculae peripherally. Usually less than 2 cm in diameter, the islands may be seen in any bone but the skull. The most frequent sites are the pelvis, femur, humerus, and ribs (1). Such lesions may be found at any age, but they are much more common in adults than in children. The lesions may appear in a bone previously documented to be normal by roentgenogram, or they may disappear after having been discovered (Fig. 10–19) (2). Bone islands are not generally believed to be active lesions, although a change in size with prolonged observation has been well documented (2). A localized area of increased uptake on bone scan, corresponding to the site of sclerotic abnormality on plain film, may be seen. Bone imaging cannot, therefore, definitively differentiate bone islands from more aggressive osseous lesions (3).

The major importance of recognizing bone islands is to distinguish them from osteoblastic metastatic lesions and osteoid osteomas. An osteoblastic metastatic lesion is usually less well defined and is not so dense as a bone island. "Thorny radiations," or a "brush border," is not seen in metastasis (4). Osteoid osteoma is usually accompanied by clinically significant

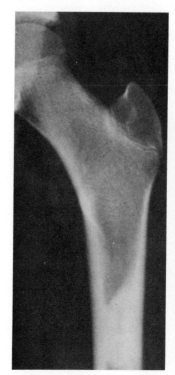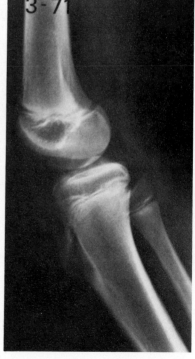

Fig. 10–19. Benign, asymptomatic bone island in femur of 13-year-old girl.

Fig. 10–20. Avulsion fracture of tibial tuberosity in 11-year-old girl.

pain, and plain film or tomography usually demonstrates a nidus within the area of sclerosis.

Histologically, bone islands or enostoses are medullary lesions composed of mature compressed lamellar bone. This bone may contain haversian systems and, therefore, resembles cortical bone. The histologic differential diagnosis involves osteoid osteoma. However, enostoses are not associated with peripheral reactive bony osteosclerosis, as is seen in an osteoid osteoma. In contrast, bone islands blend imperceptibly with the surrounding bony trabeculae.

Avulsion and Stress Fractures

Avulsion Fractures. Bony overgrowth as a response to avulsion or other trauma at growth centers may be mistaken for a neoplasm. In our experience, avulsion of the ischial and tibial tuberosities has provided the most dramatic examples (Fig. 10–20).

Devas (1) has suggested that certain types of avulsive injuries in children may be stress injuries and that many of the patients have histories suggestive of a stress fracture before the "catastrophic" avulsion.

Stress Fractures. Simple fractures, especially those classed as stress or fatigue fractures, may present difficulty in diagnosis when callus formation and periosteal reaction are seen on the roentgenogram but the underlying fracture is obscure. A healing stress fracture may simulate a primary bone tumor (usually osteogenic sarcoma) or osteomyelitis.

A history of repetitive vigorous activity associated with the onset of symptoms usually makes the diagnosis of stress fracture apparent. However, in many instances, the patient cannot recall an antecedent strenuous activity. The roentgenographic appearance of a lesion compatible with a stress fracture, in a location of common occurrence, should prompt the clinician to seek details regarding the patient's recent activities (Fig. 10–21).

Suspicion of the presence of a stress fracture despite negative findings on a plain roentgenogram should prompt a repeat examination in 1 or 2 weeks. The use of ^{99m}Tc-polyphosphate bone scanning may allow for an earlier diagnosis when a stress fracture is suspected, as the scan is usually positive before there are any roentgenographic findings (2). However, the technique is not specific for stress fracture and must be combined with a carefully taken history to establish the diagnosis.

A healing stress fracture may exhibit pronounced cellular activity, particularly in the early stages. The osteoid and chondroid material produced at this time may not be arranged in an orderly functional manner. The reparative callus results in new bone production at both the endosteal and periosteal surfaces.

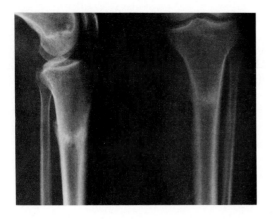

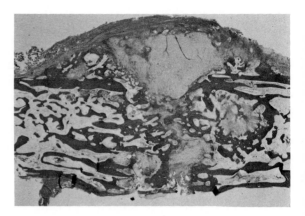

Fig. 10–21. Stress fracture in upper end of tibia in 16-year-old jogger.

Fig. 10–22. Histologically, fracture is associated with callus formation. Orderly arrangement of reactive healing response and lack of anaplasia and pleomorphism are microscopic clues to benign nature of this process. (Hematoxylin and eosin; x8.)

Most exuberant calluses that are seen in the pathology laboratory come from the ribs, but they also may come from other sites, such as the metatarsals or tibia (fatigue fracture) or pubic ramus (after total hip arthroplasty). Histologically, the cells of the callus lack nuclear atypia. The proliferating elements tend to be regularly arranged, with the earliest signs of ossification in the region adjacent to the bone and the periphery being more cellular (Fig. 10–22).

Synovial Chondromatosis

Synovial chondromatosis is a rare condition that is characterized by direct metaplasia of synovial cells into cartilage. Secondary calcification and ossification commonly occur. The lesion may originate in any focus where synovial cells are found, that is, bursae, tendon sheaths, or joints. Joint involvement is monarticular and most commonly involves the knee. Some of the metaplastic foci on the surface of the synovial membrane become sessile, then pedunculated and finally detached, producing a varying number of loose bodies (1). These bodies are subsequently nourished by the synovial fluid and may increase in size. This disorder should not be confused with other conditions that give rise to loose bodies, such as degenerative joint disease, osteochondritis dissecans, neurotrophic arthritis, and osteochondral fractures. Strict adherence to the diagnostic criteria outlined by Jaffe (2) (that is, involvement of at least 2 cm^2 of synovial membrane and formation of cartilaginous masses immediately beneath the synovial lining, with direct metaplasia and chondrocyte proliferation) is necessary to avoid confusion of this condition with other causes of loose body formation.

Synovial chondromatosis is primarily a disease of adults and is more likely to occur in males. Symptoms are usually of long duration and nonspecific (pain, swelling, and limitation of motion are most frequent) (1). In most cases, roentgenograms demonstrate multiple ossified or calcified loose bodies within the involved joint (Fig. 10–23). The joint is otherwise normal, except in long-standing disease, where secondary degenerative changes may develop. Occasionally, the loose bodies are unmineralized and the diagnosis cannot be made on the basis of roentgenographic evidence. This entity is most commonly confused with degenerative joint disease. Degenerative loose bodies tend to be larger and fewer in number, and typical degenerative changes are present in the joint.

Histologically, synovial chondromatosis presents as a lobular proliferation of cartilage within the synovium. At low-power microscopy, the synovial lining may be appreciated between the cartilaginous islands. At high magnification, however, the cytologic characteristics are worrisome for a low-grade malignant cartilage tumor (Fig. 10–24). The clinical and roentgenographic features, as well as the low-power appearance of this process, must be recognized in order to avoid an erroneous diagnosis of malignancy. This condition is almost never malignant and probably is not even a premalignant lesion.

Synovectomy, the preferred treatment, usually results in alleviation of symptoms, with a low rate of recurrence.

Massive Osteolysis

Massive osteolysis (Gorham's disease, disappearing bone disease, essential osteolysis, progressive osteolysis, phantom bone disease, spontaneous absorption of bone, vanishing bone disease, cryptogenic osteolysis) is a rare and bizarre disease characterized roentgenographically by a progressive and extensive resorption of bone and pathologically by angiomatosis.

Massive osteolysis may be confined to a single bone or may

Fig. 10–23. Synovial chondromatosis in shoulder of 24-year-old man.

Fig. 10–24. Synovial chondromatosis is histologically characterized by lobules of cartilage embedded within loose synovial connective tissue. At the periphery of these lobules, the proliferating cartilaginous tissue is hypercellular and atypical cytologic features may be identified. However, these tumors are practically never malignant. (Hematoxylin and eosin; ×16.)

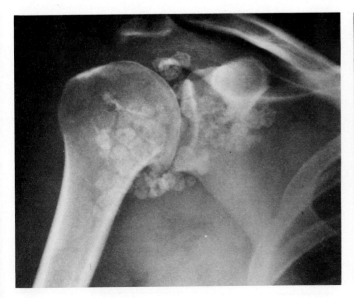

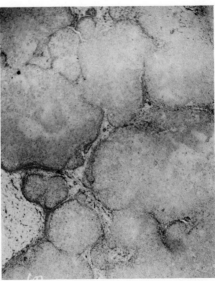

affect two or more bones centered around a joint. There appears to be a predilection for the shoulder and hip (1). In most cases, symptoms (pain, weakness, deformity, or pathologic fracture) are first noted in children or young adults, males and females being equally affected. There is usually no family history of the disease, and no endocrine or metabolic disorders have been implicated.

Despite the often relentless progression of the disease, giving the clinical impression that this phenomenon can hardly be considered anything less than "malignant," the process usually, but unpredictably, ceases.

Early during the course of the disease, roentgenograms may demonstrate intramedullary and subcortical radiolucent foci that resemble a nondescript patchy osteoporosis. When a long bone is affected, there is characteristically a concentric shrinkage of the diameter of the shaft (Fig. 10–25). No reactive sclerosis or periosteal new bone is seen. Total resorption may then follow,

Fig. 10–25. Massive osteolysis producing resorption of fifth metacarpal. Less advanced changes are present in fourth metacarpal.

Fig. 10–26. Diffuse bony involvement in mastocytosis.

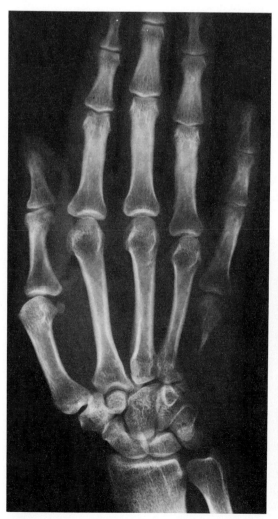

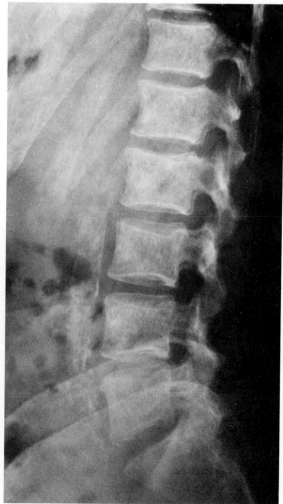

barring spontaneous arrest of the disease (2). Joints and intervertebral spaces are no barrier to extension of the process.

Histologically, massive osteolysis is characterized by cavernous angiomatous spaces. The lesion is indistinguishable from a benign hemangioma of bone, and, therefore, the diagnosis rests on clinicopathologic correlation. The endothelial cells lining the vascular spaces are flat and show no cytologic atypia. Pathologic fracture through an area of osteolysis may result in a more confusing histologic pattern because of the admixture of a healing reaction with the angioma.

This rare medical curiosity has no known cause, an unpredictable prognosis, and no known mode of therapy. Reports of successful use of radiation therapy in arresting the disease have been published, but its therapeutic value has yet to be critically evaluated.

Mastocytosis

Mastocytosis, or urticaria pigmentosa, is a rare proliferative disorder of mast cells. The skin is most often affected, producing a pruritic rash that is pigmented and urticates with minor trauma. Much less frequently, the disease may be systemic, with involvement of the liver, lymph nodes, spleen, skeleton, and gastrointestinal tract (1). Approximately half of all patients are less than 6 months old, one-fourth are adolescents, and one-fourth are adults (2). Skeletal changes occur in approximately 10% of patients with urticaria pigmentosa and approximately 70% with systemic mastocytosis (2).

The roentgenographic manifestation may be localized, consisting of a few scattered slightly irregular patches of increased density or oval radiolucencies surrounded by a sclerotic halo. Most frequently involved are the skull, vertebrae, pelvis, and ends of long bones. In other patients, bony involvement is diffuse and widespread throughout the skeleton and is not sharply demarcated from the surrounding bone. Osteosclerotic changes are prominent, intermingled with osteoporosis. This spotty admixture gives the skeleton an appearance that may be easily confused with metastatic carcinoma (Fig. 10–26). In contrast to metastatic lesions, however, truly destructive lesions are not seen in mastocytosis and the bones are not weakened, so that pathologic fractures do not occur. The lytic areas with sclerotic halos have a smooth reactive rather than an indistinct margin.

In most instances, the suspicion of mastocytosis may be confirmed by detection of the characteristic skin lesions or the frequent mild to moderate hepatosplenomegaly. Bone biopsy may assure the correct diagnosis, although the number of mast cells in a given specimen may not be increased (1).

Biopsy specimens of bone in mastocytosis characteristically show a small-cell infiltrate (Fig. 10–27). On low-power microscopy, the cellular infiltrate may have a granuloma-like appearance and may be associated with fibrosis of the marrow. The

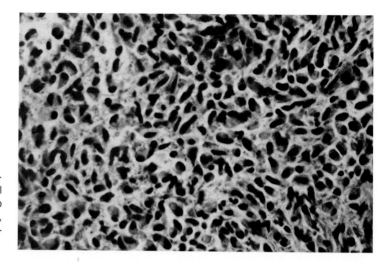

Fig. 10–27. Bony lesions of mastocytosis are histologically composed of small cells which may show some tendency to spindle or form granuloma-like masses, as in this case involving the ilium. (Hematoxylin and eosin; ×1,400.)

bony trabeculae may show sclerosis, resulting in a pagetoid appearance. Special stains (Giemsa) can be used to document the metachromatic cytoplasmic granules found in mast cells. However, bony lesions that have been subject to decalcification generally will show only a few granules. Therefore, if mastocytosis is suspected, bony lesions should be carefully examined at high magnification for cytoplasmic granules. Metachromatic granules are more easily identified in skin lesions. A high index of suspicion and collaborative clinical information are necessary in order to diagnose confidently mastocytosis in bony lesions.

Fibrous Dysplasia

Fibrous dysplasia is probably a developmental abnormality characterized by fibrous replacement of portions of the medullary cavities of a bone or bones. Patches of yellow or brown skin pigmentation with an irregular ("coast of Maine") contour may accompany the bone lesions, usually in patients with severe, widespread disease. When typical skin lesions are associated with polyostotic disease and endocrine abnormalities, especially precocious puberty in the female, the condition is called Albright's syndrome.

Both sexes are affected equally. The disease begins in young persons, often in infancy, but many of the bony lesions are completely asymptomatic and are unrecognized. Limp, pain in an extremity, or pathologic fracture is the usual presenting symptom (1). Leg-length discrepancy, most often the result of a shepherd's crook deformity of the proximal femur, is the most common physical finding. One also may detect bowing of the tibia or rib deformities (1).

Adult patients with polyostotic disease are sometimes considered to have hyperparathyroidism on the basis of the initial findings on the roentgenographic examination (2). Solitary lesions may be mistaken for true neoplasia, and treatment is more vigorous than necessary. Monostotic disease also may be confused with nonossifying fibroma, unicameral bone cyst, and even aneurysmal bone cyst. A thorough familiarity with the roentgenographic features of fibrous dysplasia usually will allow a correct diagnosis.

Monostotic fibrous dysplasia has a varied, but often characteristic, roentgenographic appearance. The lesions originate within the medullary portion of the bone, most commonly in the metaphysis. The density varies from completely radiolucent to a "ground-glass" appearance, a homogeneously increased density (Fig. 10–28). In the lesions with increased density, the distinction between cortex and medulla may be lost. Monostotic fibrous dysplasia has a benign appearance and often a dense sclerotic margin. Endosteal erosion and expansion are often present. Periosteal new bone is not present in uncomplicated lesions. Occasionally, it may be impossible to distinguish solitary lesions of fibrous dysplasia from other benign bone lesions, such as unicameral bone cyst and nonossifying fibroma.

Fibrous dysplasia may affect any bone, but it is most commonly found when the jaw or base of the skull is involved. Grossly, these lesions are firm and may be gritty because of osteoid trabeculae. Histologically, the lesions are an admixture of benign proliferating fibroblastic cells and islands of woven bone. The bony trabeculae are characteristically arranged in a haphazard fashion (Fig. 10–29). Benign giant cells and macrophages are commonly associated with degenerative foci.

Treatment should be conservative and aimed at prevention of deformity. Many but not all lesions stop growing at puberty. Surgery should be considered for significant or progressive deformity, pain unresponsive to conservative management, and impending pathologic fracture. Curettage and bone grafting is usually successful, although recurrence may be troublesome.

There are numerous reports of sarcomatous degeneration in the literature. Many of these patients have been previously treated with radiation therapy (3–5).

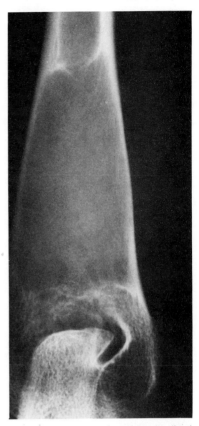

Fig. 10–28. Fibrous dysplasia in distal humeral metaphysis.

Osteofibrous Dysplasia

Osteofibrous dysplasia is now recognized as a distinct clinicopathologic entity that had previously been mistaken for fibrous dysplasia. It occurs almost exclusively in the tibia and fibula and is distinct from fibrous dysplasia with respect to patient age, roentgenographic appearance, histologic features, and clinical course.

Campanacci (1) originally described this entity and noted that previous authors had reported similar cases under the following diagnoses: congenital fibrous dysplasia, fibrous dysplasia associated with tibial curvature, infantile pseudarthrosis of the tibia, congenital fibrous defect of the tibia, and ossifying fibroma.

Osteofibrous dysplasia, having a slight predilection for males, always occurs within the first 10 years of life, most often within

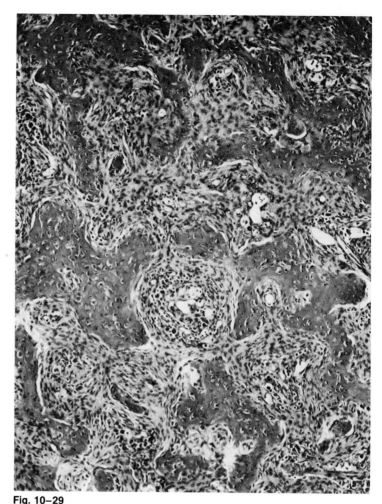

Fig. 10–29

Fig. 10–29. The presence of trabeculae arranged in haphazard fashion among benign fibroblastic proliferation is characteristic of fibrous dysplasia. (Hematoxylin and eosin; ×100.)

Fig. 10–30. Osteofibrous dysplasia of tibia.

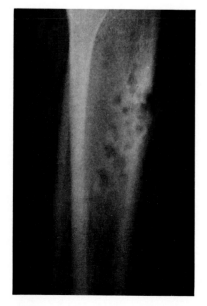

the first 5 years. The usual presenting complaint is enlargement of the tibia, often associated with slight or moderate anterior bowing. Pathologic fractures and pseudarthroses are less commonly encountered. The lesion is typically diaphyseal, involving the middle third of the tibia. Fibular lesions are always in the distal third.

Tibial lesions are characterized roentgenographically by their eccentric and usually anterior locations within the tibial shaft (Fig. 10–30). Single or multiple lucent areas are surrounded by dense sclerosis, which is thickest internally. The medullary canal is frequently narrowed at the site of involvement. Anterior bowing of the tibial shaft is common and well demonstrated on roentgenograms. The roentgenographic appearance closely resembles and may be identical to that of adamantinoma. The age of the patient is the most important distinguishing feature.

Grossly, the cortex remains intact over the region of osteofibrous dysplasia. The underlying lesion varies from yellow to red and from soft to firm. Histologically, the lesion mimics fibrous dysplasia, with bony trabeculae scattered through a fibrous stroma. However, in contrast to fibrous dysplasia, the bony trabeculae are bordered by osteoblasts. Toward the center of the lesion, the fibrous tissue may be looser, and foci simulating nonossifying fibroma also may be identified within the lesion.

The prognosis is favorable, more so than in fibrous dysplasia. There is little tendency to progression in patients who are more than 5 years old. Some lesions heal spontaneously. Excision or resection is likely to be followed by recurrence and should not be attempted early in the course of the disease. When the patient is 5 years old, surgery should be considered only for patients with lesions that are large enough to make pathologic fracture imminent. However, such fractures will heal spontaneously with simple immobilization. If indicated, correction of residual bowing with one or multiple osteotomies should be delayed until the patient is 10 to 12 years old.

Histiocytosis X

Histiocytosis X includes the entities of eosinophilic granuloma, Hand-Schüller-Christian disease, and Letterer-Siwe disease. Despite their common histopathologic appearance (Fig. 10–31), there is a continuing debate as to whether these three clinical diseases are variable manifestations of a single pathologic process (1). The cause of the histiocytosis is still not understood. No evidence of a metabolic or lipid-storage disease exists, and there is no characteristic hereditary pattern. Based on the nature of the disease, a viral etiology has been frequently proposed, but a specific agent has not been identified.

Eosinophilic granuloma is a disease in which single and occasionally multiple bones are involved, with no extraskeletal involvement. The highest incidence is during the first three decades of life, and the disease is most common in patients who are between 5 and 10 years old. The prognosis is good, and the disease is usually curable. Hand-Schüller-Christian disease (chronic disseminated histiocytosis) is marked by both skeletal and visceral involvement. The onset is characteristically seen in children between 5 and 10 years of age, but some patients have had the onset from birth through the fifth decade. The disease has a chronic course, and the prognosis depends on the degree of involvement and the age at onset. Letterer-Siwe disease is an acute and fulminant disease that affects infants and young children who are less than 2 years old. The patients are extremely ill, and the prognosis is very poor.

The underlying disease process in this group of conditions may evoke a diffuse variety of clinical signs and symptoms. Patients with eosinophilic granuloma usually present with complaints of pain limited to the local area of skeletal involvement. There may be tenderness or warmth at the site of the lesion. Patients less than 20 years old have the skull and femur most frequently involved, whereas those more than 20 years old have

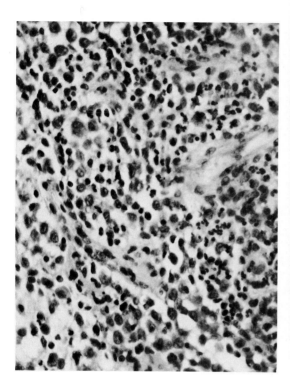

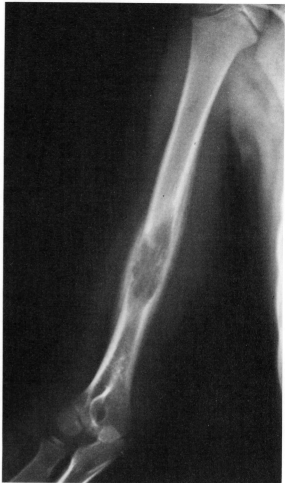

Fig. 10–31. Histologically, lesions of eosinophilic granuloma, Hand-Schüller-Christian disease, and Letterer-Siwe disease are similar. A mixed inflammatory infiltrate, often including numerous eosinophils, accompanies the "sheet-like" infiltrate of histiocytes with their characteristic grooved nuclear contours. (Hematoxylin and eosin; x400.)

Fig. 10–32. Histiocytosis X in humeral shaft with smooth periosteal new bone.

the ribs and mandible most frequently involved (2). Vertebral lesions may be manifested by local pain, stiffness, and occasionally neurologic findings.

Hand-Schüller-Christian disease may involve multiple organ systems in addition to bone, producing protean clinical expressions related to involvement of these organ systems. The classic triad of exophthalmos, diabetes insipidus, and rarefied defects of bone of the skull probably occurs in less than 10% of patients (3). A partial triad, however, has equal significance if other evidences of dissemination such as anemia, splenomegaly, fatigability, loss of weight, and lymphadenopathy are present (4). Involvement of the integument results in yellow nodules or plaques on the skin or ulcers on the palate, gums, or vulva. Involvement of the sphenoid bone is reputed to cause pituitary dysfunction in approximately one-third of the patients, although the exact pathologic mechanism is unknown. Exophthalmos occurs from retro-orbital invasion. Discharge from the ears (chronic serous otitis) results from involvement of the petrous portion of the temporal bone. Jaw involvement may eventuate in loose teeth or even loss of teeth.

The roentgenographic appearance of the skeletal lesions is similar in all the clinical forms of histiocytosis X. Radiolucent bone defects occur in any portion of the involved bone and may cause endosteal scalloping and expansion. The type of bone destruction is most commonly geographic, rather than permeative or moth-eaten. Uneven destruction of cortical surfaces or the tables of the skull produces beveling and a "hole-within-a-hole" appearance. Reactive marginal sclerosis may be seen, especially after therapy. Periosteal new bone is common and usually appears solid and benign (Fig. 10–32). In the spinal column, either uniform or asymmetrical flattening of vertebral bodies may be seen. Skeletal lesions in adults are often much more sclerotic than those seen in children.

Typical skull lesions, polyostotic involvement, and vertebra plana are all suggestive of the diagnosis. Individual lesions also may be characteristic, but biopsy is often necessary for diagnosis and differentiation from osteomyelitis or even Ewing's sarcoma.

Classically, treatment for eosinophilic granuloma has been surgery or radiation therapy. A symptomatic solitary lesion that is surgically accessible is managed by curettage and bone grafting, when the structural integrity of the involved part has been compromised. The recurrence rate is low. When multiple lesions are present, a period of observation (as long as 1 year or more) for patients with nonsymptomatic lesions may permit spontaneous healing (5). Low-dose radiation (300 to 600 rads) may be given to those lesions that do not require surgery and that are asymptomatic. Recently, Cohen et al. (6) reported on a series of patients treated by the direct injection of methylprednisolone acetate into the lesion and have obtained encouraging results.

Treatment of Hand-Schüller-Christian disease and Letterer-Siwe disease is more complex. In addition to surgery (usually limited to a specific area of bony involvement which is symptomatic or has undergone pathologic fracture), systemic corticosteroids or chemotherapy may be utilized (7).

Heterotopic Ossification

Localized areas of active myositis ossificans, occurring with or without a definite history of antecedent trauma, may be mistaken both roentgenographically and pathologically for a malignancy. According to Ackerman (1), heterotopic ossification is a preferable designation over myositis ossificans for this lesion, as "there is no inflammation, often no bone, and in some instances muscle is not included in the pathological process" (1).

Heterotopic bone formation occurs as a result of a single episode of trauma or of repetitive minor trauma. However,

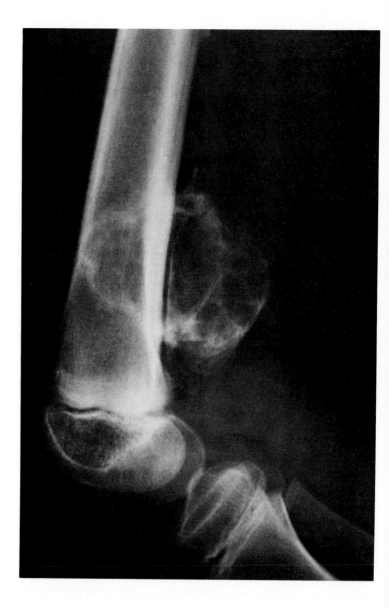

Fig. 10–33. Heterotopic ossification in thigh of 9-year-old girl who had fallen 3 months before the roentgenogram was taken.

many patients present without a history of injury. It may be that injury has occurred but that it was so slight as to have gone unrecognized. Some authors have referred to localized lesions of heterotopic ossification in which there is no history of antecedent trauma as "pseudomalignant osseous tumors of soft tissue." Frequent sites of this lesion include the anterior aspect of the thigh, upper arm (brachialis anticus most frequently), adductor muscles, and gluteal muscles. Usually, the earliest physical finding is that of a doughy mass present several hours after injury.

Early during the course of the condition, roentgenograms will show no abnormality or only a nondescript soft-tissue mass. Ossification first becomes visible within the mass 2 to 3 weeks after the injury. At this stage, the roentgenographic appearance may be suggestive of a soft-tissue sarcoma. A lucent zone clearly separates the ossification from the underlying bone. Smooth, benign-appearing periosteal new bone may form on the underlying bone, but the cortex itself is normal. During the second month, the heterotopic ossification begins to mature and develops a characteristic peripheral rim of dense ossification (Fig. 10–33). The rapid evolution of this lesion within the first few weeks is distinctive, and serial films are often helpful if the diagnosis is in doubt. As the heterotopic bone matures during the subsequent months and years, it becomes smaller and often fuses with the underlying bone to form an exostosis.

Grossly, the lesions of heterotopic ossification tend to be well circumscribed, except in their early stages of development. Most commonly, the origin of this process away from bone is obvious; however, similar reactive processes may occur on the surface of bone involving the periosteum. Histologically, these lesions show a characteristic maturation to benign osteocartilaginous components at the periphery. However, in their early stage of development and at the center of more mature lesions, there may be mitotically active foci with cytologic atypia. This zoning phenomenon is helpful in the histologic identification of this process (Fig. 10–34).

On the assumption that the lesion has been correctly identified, no treatment is usually necessary. As Dahlin has pointed out, "The prognosis is good whether the lesion is excised or amputation is performed because of an erroneous diagnosis" (2). Should excision of a large mass causing pain or limitation of function be contemplated, surgical intervention should be delayed until serial roentgenograms have demonstrated the lesion to be dense, well demarcated, and without growth. Most lesions, however, will spontaneously regress with time.

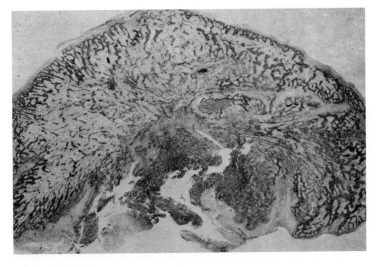

Fig. 10–34. Low-power photomicrograph of soft-tissue lesion from forearm shows characteristic "zoning" phenomenon characteristic of myositis ossificans or heterotopic ossification. Toward the periphery of the lesion, the bony trabeculae are well formed and arranged in parallel arrays. Cytologically, the proliferating cells lack anaplastic features. (Hematoxylin and eosin; x60.)

Lesions Simulating Tumors of Bone

References
UNICAMERAL BONE CYST

1. Morton KS: The pathogenesis of unicameral bone cyst. Can J Surg 7:140–150, 1964
2. Jaffe HL, Lichtenstein L: Solitary unicameral bone cyst with emphasis on the roentgen picture, the pathologic appearance and the pathogenesis. Arch Surg 44:1004–1025, 1942
3. Cohen J: Unicameral bone cysts: a current synthesis of reported cases. Orthop Clin North Am 8:715–736, 1977
4. Boseker EH, Bickel WH, Dahlin DC: A clinicopathologic study of simple unicameral bone cysts. Surg Gynecol Obstet 127:550–560, 1968
5. Neer CS, Francis KC, Marcove RC, et al: Treatment of unicameral bone cyst: a follow-up study of one hundred seventy-five cases. J Bone Joint Surg [Am] 48:731–745, 1966
6. Scaglietti O, Marchetti PG, Bartolozzi P: The effects of methylprednisolone acetate in the treatment of bone cysts: results of three years follow-up. J Bone Joint Surg [Br] 61:200–204, 1979
7. Smith RW, Smith CF: Solitary unicameral bone cyst of the calcaneus: a review of twenty cases. J Bone Joint Surg [Am] 56:49–56, 1974
8. Abe M, Iwakura H, Ohno T, et al: Solitary bone cyst of the calcaneus. J Jpn Orthop Assoc 51:171–180, 1977

ANEURYSMAL BONE CYST

1. Tillman BP, Dahlin DC, Lipscomb PR, et al: Aneurysmal bone cyst: an analysis of ninety-five cases. Mayo Clin Proc 43:478–495, 1968
2. Dahlin DC: Bone Tumors: General Aspects and Data on 6,221 Cases. Third edition. Springfield, Illinois, Charles C Thomas, Publisher, 1978
3. Nobler MP, Higinbotham NL, Phillips RF: The cure of aneurysmal bone cyst: irradiation superior to surgery in an analysis of 33 cases. Radiology 90:1185–1192, 1968

CYSTS ASSOCIATED WITH DISEASES OF JOINTS

1. Hunder GG, Ward LE, Ivins JC: Rheumatoid granulomatous lesion simulating malignancy in the head and neck of the femur. Mayo Clin Proc 40:766–770, 1965
2. Dahlin DC: Bone Tumors: General Aspects and Data on 6,221 Cases. Third edition. Springfield, Illinois, Charles C Thomas, Publisher, 1978

GANGLION CYSTS OF BONE

1. Sim FH, Dahlin DC: Ganglion cysts of bone. Mayo Clin Proc 46:484–488, 1971
2. Kambolis C, Bullough PG, Jaffe HL: Ganglionic cystic defects of bone. J Bone Joint Surg [Am] 55:496–505, 1973
3. Feldman F, Johnston AD: Ganglia of bone: theories, manifestations, and presentations. CRC Crit Rev Clin Radiol Nucl Med 4:303–332, 1973

PSEUDOCYSTS OF HUMERUS

1. Helms CA: Pseudocysts of the humerus. AJR 131:287–288, 1978

OSTEOMYELITIS

1. Elliott GR: Chronic osteomyelitis presenting distinct tumor formation simulating clinically true osteogenic sarcoma. J Bone Joint Surg 16:137–144, 1934
2. Cabanela ME, Sim FH, Beabout JW, et al: Osteomyelitis appearing as neoplasms: a diagnostic problem. Arch Surg 109:68–72, 1974

3. Dahlin DC: Bone Tumors: General Aspects and Data on 6,221 Cases. Third edition. Springfield, Illinois, Charles C Thomas, Publisher, 1978

HYPERPARATHYROIDISM

1. Edeiken J: Roentgen Diagnosis of Diseases of Bone. Vol. I. Third edition. Baltimore, Williams & Wilkins Company, 1981
2. Dahlin DC: Bone Tumors: General Aspects and Data on 6,221 Cases. Third edition. Springfield, Illinois, Charles C Thomas, Publisher, 1978
3. Lichtenstein L: Bone Tumors. Fourth edition. St Louis, CV Mosby Company, 1972

PAGET'S DISEASE OF BONE

1. Lichtenstein L: Bone Tumors. Fourth edition. St Louis, CV Mosby Company, 1972
2. Dahlin DC: Bone Tumors: General Aspects and Data on 6,221 Cases. Third edition. Springfield, Illinois, Charles C Thomas, Publisher, 1978

AVULSIVE CORTICAL IRREGULARITY

1. Barnes GR Jr, Gwinn JL: Distal irregularities of the femur simulating malignancy. Am J Roentgenol 122:180–185, 1974
2. Kimmelstiel P, Rapp I: Cortical defect due to periosteal desmoids. Bull Hosp Joint Dis 12:286–297, 1951
3. Bufkin WJ: The avulsive cortical irregularity. Am J Roentgenol Radium Ther Nucl Med 112:487–492, 1971
4. Simon H: Medial distal metaphyseal femoral irregularity in children. Radiology 90:258–260, 1968
5. Young DW, Nogrady MB, Dunbar JS, et al: Benign cortical irregularities in the distal femur of children. J Can Assoc Radiol 23:107–115, 1972
6. Edeiken J: Roentgen Diagnosis of Diseases of Bone. Vol. I. Third edition. Baltimore, Williams & Wilkins Company, 1981, p 116

BONE INFARCTS

1. Bullough PG, Kambolis CP, Marcove RC, et al: Bone infarctions not associated with caisson disease. J Bone Joint Surg [Am] 47:477–491, 1965
2. Dahlin DC: Bone Tumors: General Aspects and Data on 6,221 Cases. Third edition. Springfield, Illinois, Charles C Thomas, Publisher, 1978
3. Furey JG, Ferrer-Torells M, Reagan JW: Fibrosarcoma arising at the site of bone infarcts: a report of two cases. J Bone Joint Surg [Am]42:802–810, 1960

BONE ISLANDS

1. Edeiken J: Roentgen Diagnosis of Diseases of Bone. Vol. I. Third edition. Baltimore, Williams & Wilkins Company, 1981
2. Onitsuka H: Roentgenologic aspects of bone islands. Radiology 123:607–612, 1977
3. Kim SK, Barry WF Jr: Bone islands. Radiology 90:77–78, 1969
4. Davies JAK, Hall FM, Goldberg RP, et al: Positive bone scan in a bone island: case report. J Bone Joint Surg [Am] 61:943–945, 1979

AVULSION AND STRESS FRACTURES

1. Devas M: Stress Fractures. New York, Churchill Livingstone, 1975, pp 190–211
2. Wilcox JR Jr, Moniot AL, Green JP: Bone scanning in the evaluation of exercise-related stress injuries. Radiology 123:699–703, 1977

SYNOVIAL CHONDROMATOSIS

1. Murphy FP, Dahlin DC, Sullivan CR: Articular synovial chondromatosis. J Bone Joint Surg [Am] 44:77–86, 1962
2. Jaffe HL: Synovial chondromatosis and other benign articular tumors. *In* Tumors and Tumorous Conditions of the Bones and Joints. Philadelphia, Lea & Febiger, 1958, pp 558–575

MASSIVE OSTEOLYSIS

1. Bullough PG: Massive osteolysis. NY State J Med 71:2267–2278, 1971
2. Johnson PM, McClure JG: Observations on massive osteolysis: a review of the literature and report of a case. Radiology 71:28–41, 1958

MASTOCYTOSIS

1. Barer M, Peterson LF, Dahlin DC, et al: Mastocytosis with osseous lesions resembling metastatic malignant lesions of bone. J Bone Joint Surg [Am] 50:142–152, 1968
2. Sagher F, Even-Paz Z: Mastocytosis and the Mast Cell. Chicago, Year Book Medical Publishers, 1967

FIBROUS DYSPLASIA

1. Harris WH, Dudley HR Jr, Barry RJ: The natural history of fibrous dysplasia: an orthopaedic, pathological, and roentgenographic study. J Bone Joint Surg [Am] 44:207–233, 1962
2. Lichtenstein L: Bone Tumors. Fourth edition. St Louis, CV Mosby Company, 1972
3. Coley BL, Stewart FW: Bone sarcoma in polyostotic fibrous dysplasia. Ann Surg 121:872–881, 1945
4. Perkinson NG, Higinbotham NL: Osteogenic sarcoma arising in polyostotic fibrous dysplasia: report of a case. Cancer 8:396–402, 1955
5. Schwartz DT, Alpert M: The malignant transformation of fibrous dysplasia. Am J Med Sci 247:1–20, 1964

OSTEOFIBROUS DYSPLASIA

1. Campanacci M: Osteofibrous dysplasia of long bones: a new clinical entity. Ital J Orthop Traumatol 2:221–237, 1976

HISTIOCYTOSIS X

1. Lichtenstein L: Histiocytosis X: integration of eosinophilic granuloma of bone, "Letterer-Siwe disease," and "Schüller-Christian disease" as related manifestations of a single nosologic entity. Arch Pathol 56:84–102, 1953
2. Schajowicz F, Slullitel J: Eosinophilic granuloma of bone and its relationship to Hand-Schüller-Christian and Letterer-Siwe syndromes. J Bone Joint Surg [Br] 55:545–565, 1973
3. Lichtenstein L: Histiocytosis X (eosinophilic granuloma of bone, Letterer-Siwe disease, and Schüller-Christian disease): further observations of pathological and clinical importance. J Bone Joint Surg [Am] 46:76–90, 1964
4. Dahlin DC: Bone Tumors: General Aspects and Data on 6,221 Cases. Third edition. Springfield, Illinois, Charles C Thomas, Publisher, 1978
5. Mickelson MR, Bonfiglio M: Eosinophilic granuloma and its variations. Orthop Clin North Am 8:933–945, 1977
6. Cohen M, Zornoza J, Cangir A, et al: Direct injection of methylprednisolone sodium succinate in the treatment of solitary eosinophilic granuloma of bone: a report of 9 cases. Radiology 136:289–293, 1980
7. Winkelmann RK, Burgert EO: Therapy of histiocytosis X. Br J Dermatol 82:169–175, 1970

HETEROTOPIC OSSIFICATION

1. Ackerman LV: Extra-osseous localized non-neoplastic bone and cartilage formation (so-called myositis ossificans): clinical and pathological
   confusion with malignant neoplasms. J Bone Joint Surg [Am] 40:279–
   298, 1958
2. Dahlin DC: Bone Tumors: General Aspects and Data on 6,221 Cases.
   Third edition. Springfield, Illinois, Charles C Thomas, Publisher, 1978

Section III:

Malignant Tumors

CHAPTER 11

OSTEOSARCOMA AND ITS VARIANTS

Douglas J. Pritchard, M.D.
David C. Dahlin, M.D.
John H. Edmonson, M.D.

Osteosarcoma is the most common primary bone sarcoma, accounting for about 20% of all bone sarcomas. The definition of osteosarcoma utilized by Lichtenstein (1) is accepted by most bone pathologists. Histologic diagnosis requires (1) the presence of a frankly sarcomatous stroma and (2) the direct formation of tumor osteoid and bone by this malignant connective tissue. Since there is no definitive way of recognizing osteoid even by special stains, it is sometimes difficult to be certain of the histologic diagnosis. The microscopic appearance of osteoid is similar to that of collagen and cartilage matrix, so that on occasion the histopathologic diagnosis may be somewhat arbitrary. However, in situations in which the presence of osteoid is equivocal, clinical features and the roentgenographic appearance of the lesion may be helpful in arriving at a definitive diagnosis. The problem is even more complex because there are a number of different variants of classic osteosarcoma, each of which may have its own distinctive clinical and biologic behavior (2) (Table 11-1). Each of these variants must be considered when one is classifying and analyzing the results of various clinical trials.

Clinical Features

Classic osteosarcoma tends to occur in teenagers and young adults. Paget's disease is a known precursor of osteosarcoma. Since Paget's disease occurs in older adults, if there is a large population of patients with Paget's disease, there may be a secondary peak in the incidence of osteosarcoma in later years. In Great Britain, for example, where Paget's disease is much more prevalent than it is in the United States, there is a secondary peak—at 50 to 60 years of age—in the incidence of osteosarcoma. As do most other bone tumors, osteosarcomas commonly afflict more males than females (Fig. 11-1). About half of all osteosarcomas occur in the region of the knee joint, the distal femur being the most frequent location. Osteosarcoma tends to occur in the metaphyseal region of a long bone; when the physis is still present, the tumor tends to remain in the

Table 11—1.—Types of Osteosarcoma

"Usual" osteosarcoma
  In jaws
  In Paget's disease
  Telangiectatic
  Malignant fibrous histiocytoma
  Periosteal
  In other benign lesions
  Multicentric
  Low-grade, central
Parosteal osteosarcoma
Postirradiation sarcoma
Dedifferentiated chondrosarcoma

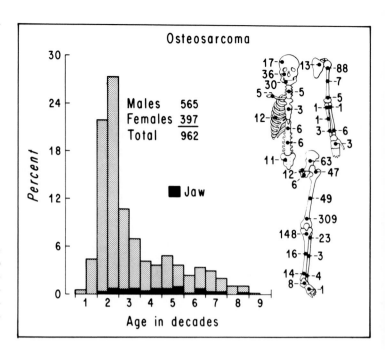

Fig. 11-1. Skeletal, age, and sex distribution of osteosarcomas at the Mayo Clinic. (From Dahlin DC, Unni KK: Osteosarcoma of bone and its important recognizable varieties. Am J Surg Pathol 1:61-72, 1977. By permission of Masson Publishing USA, Inc.)

metaphysis without crossing into the epiphysis. There are exceptions, however, as when the lesion may be located entirely within the epiphysis. In addition, diaphyseal lesions and lesions of the flat bones are not uncommon. Osteosarcomas that occur in the jaw bones represent a special group because the clinical behavior of osteosarcoma in this location is different.

As do most bone tumors, osteosarcomas produce nonspecific symptoms. Most patients complain of pain or a mass or both. Patients with osteosarcoma usually do not present with a pathologic fracture. Symptoms are generally present for several months before the diagnosis is established; patients with classic osteosarcoma usually do not have symptoms for more than a year before diagnosis. Patients who have symptoms present for a prolonged period may have a better prognosis than those who are seen soon after the symptoms are apparent. This difference may reflect the aggressiveness of the particular tumor. For patients with some underlying condition such as Paget's disease or prior radiation for some other condition, a change in symptoms may herald the development of malignant transformation.

There is considerable current interest in relating laboratory findings to the diagnosis and prognosis of osteosarcoma. The serum alkaline phosphatase level, which indicates osteoblastic activity, may be greatly elevated in the normal growing child. This elevation makes the interpretation of the serum alkaline phosphatase level in teenagers difficult and its usefulness, therefore, obscured. In adults, however, an elevated alkaline phosphatase level may have prognostic importance. There are no laboratory tests that aid in the diagnosis. However, several experimental approaches currently are being investigated which may be helpful in establishing the prognosis. One such example is the tissue level of alkaline phosphatase: preliminary studies indicate that higher tumor levels of alkaline phosphatase indicate a worse prognosis.

There are no characteristic physical findings with classic osteosarcoma. Many patients have extraskeletal extension of the lesion and therefore may have a palpable mass. There may be increased warmth or dilated subcutaneous veins overlying the tumor.

Roentgenographic Findings

Osteosarcoma usually is seen as a destructive lesion with indistinct borders that gradually merge into the adjacent normal bone. While some small tumors may be entirely within medullary bone, osteosarcoma generally extends into the cortex or even breaks through the cortex into the surrounding soft tissues. Various amounts of calcification and mineralized bone are usually present within the lesion. In addition, periosteal new bone formation may be evident at the periphery of the lesion. The bone within the tumor tends to be streaked and have a "sunburst" appearance. No one feature, however, is common to this tumor. The roentgenographic appearance of osteosarcoma may vary considerably. A tumor that is mostly osteoblastic may have large areas of sclerotic bone with a fairly characteristic appearance (Fig. 11-2 A). If the tumor is primarily telangiectatic, the entire lesion may appear to be cystic; the roentgenographic appearance of a telangiectatic osteosarcoma may be indistinguishable from that of an aneurysmal bone cyst or even a benign giant cell tumor (Fig. 11-2 B).

Parosteal osteosarcoma is a rare tumor that seems to arise from the surface of bone and has distinctive roentgenographic and histologic features and a relatively benign clinical course (Fig. 11-2 C). Periosteal osteosarcoma, sometimes referred to as juxtacortical chondrosarcoma, is another rare tumor with a fairly characteristic roentgenographic appearance. The histologic and biologic features of this neoplasm are distinctly different from those of an ordinary or clinically apparent osteosarcoma (Fig. 11-3 A). The low-grade central variety of osteosarcoma has a more indolent roentgenographic appearance than does the classic osteosarcoma. This lesion may be confused with fibrous dysplasia (Fig. 11-3 B).

Pathologic Findings

Gross. Most osteosarcomas are relatively large, with extension through cortical bone and into the adjacent soft tissues. The tumor may vary in consistency from areas that are densely sclerotic to areas that are very soft or fibrous. Generally, the central portion is sclerotic and the most peripheral portion is soft. This difference may be important when taking a biopsy specimen because the soft peripheral portion not only is easier to approach and to process in the pathology laboratory but also is more likely to be the most malignant portion of the tumor. There may be cystic areas and areas of necrosis, especially in large tumors. The tumor also tends to extend within the medullary canal in any direction. Enneking and Kagan (3) noted skip areas within the medullary canal—that is, areas of tumor without intervening extension of the tumor. Such areas presumably represent metastasis within the medullary canal and may indicate that the prognosis is particularly poor.

Microscopic. The histologic appearance of classic osteosarcoma may vary considerably. Osteoid tissue, chondroid tissue, and fibrinoid tissue may be present in various amounts. Often, one of these elements predominates; this allows one to categorize these lesions as osteoblastic, chondroblastic, or fibroblastic (4) (Fig. 11-4). Some lesions have a mixture of two or more elements, and it is not possible to determine which element predominates. All osteosarcomas, however, have osteoid. It may be difficult to demonstrate osteoid, and considerable expertise and judgment is often necessary to establish its presence. Because benign lesions may provoke an osteoid response, the mere presence of osteoid is not indicative of osteosarcoma. Rather, osteoid should be considered as being produced by the adjacent sarcomatous cells. Again, reliable interpretation of the histologic findings requires an experienced pathologist. Rarely, it may be exceedingly difficult to differentiate a chondroblastic osteosarcoma from a chondrosarcoma.

The cells of osteosarcoma may vary considerably in size, shape, and degree of anaplasia. Benign-appearing giant cells may be encountered. Because cells in the central portion of the tumor may be smaller than cells in the periphery, the degree of anaplasia in the central portion may be less apparent. Frequently, the cells are dispersed in a lacelike stroma of osteoid; in some lesions, however, the osteoid is not so obvious, and multiple sections may be required before the presence of osteoid is established.

In addition to differentiating the histologic subtypes of osteosarcoma, a microscopic grade usually can be established according to the method of Broders. Most osteosarcomas are high-grade anaplastic lesions. However, lower-grade lesions are sometimes encountered. Grade I osteosarcoma may have only subtle evidence of malignancy. Again, it must be emphasized that while some osteosarcomas are relatively easy to diagnose, others may be extremely difficult, even for the experienced bone pathologist.

Metastases. Osteosarcoma tends to metastasize to the lungs. In general, these metastatic lesions occur on the periphery of

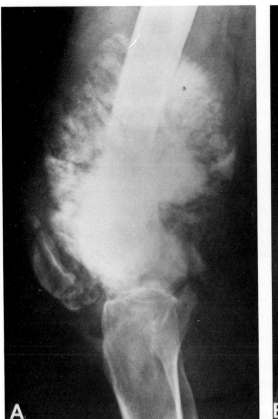

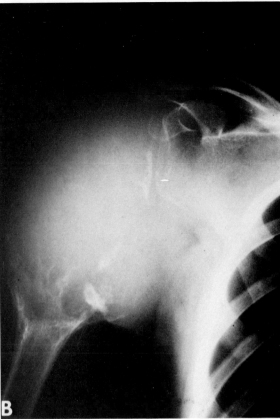

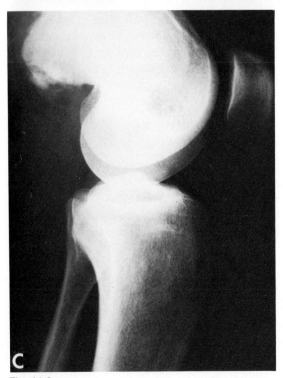

Fig. 11-2. *A*, Large, high-grade osteo-blastic osteosarcoma arising in distal femur of an adult. *B*, Telangiectatic osteosarcoma of proximal humerus, almost totally lytic. *C*, Parosteal osteosarcoma arising from posterior surface of distal femur.

Fig. 11-2.

Osteosarcoma and Its Variants

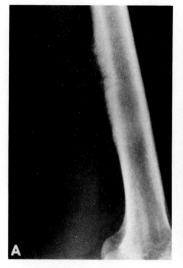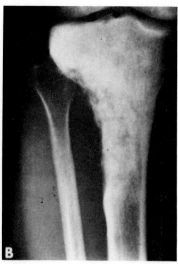

Fig. 11-3. *A,* Periosteal osteosarcoma arising from surface of femur; characteristic roentgenologic appearance. *B,* low-grade, central osteosarcoma of tibia. Lesion was present for several years before diagnosis.

the lung fields rather than within the lung parenchyma. When metastasis occurs, it usually does so within the first 2 years after the original definitive treatment. However, metastasis may occur many years later. In the absence of pulmonary metastasis, metastasis rarely occurs to other bones. When this occurs, the condition is referred to as metachronous osteosarcoma. When multiple bones are involved at the outset, the condition is referred to as multicentric osteosarcoma. Other organs may be involved with metastatic disease, but only rarely does this happen without pulmonary metastasis occurring first.

Treatment

Preoperative Evaluation. In addition to the usual careful history, physical examination, and routine laboratory tests, several other examinations are very helpful. The radioisotopic bone scan using technetium-99 is valuable, both in ruling out the possibility of other bony lesions and in determining the precise extent of the primary tumor. Occasionally, even pulmonary metastatic lesions will be apparent on the bone scan. Localized tomograms are occasionally helpful in determining the extent of the primary tumor. These may be particularly useful when a lesion appears to have a periosteal origin. Sometimes such a lesion tends to surround the bone, making it impossible to determine by plain roentgenograms whether the medullary canal is involved. If a parosteal osteosarcoma extends into the medullary canal, its clinical behavior will be more like that of classic osteosarcoma than of an ordinary parosteal osteosarcoma. This

Bone Tumors

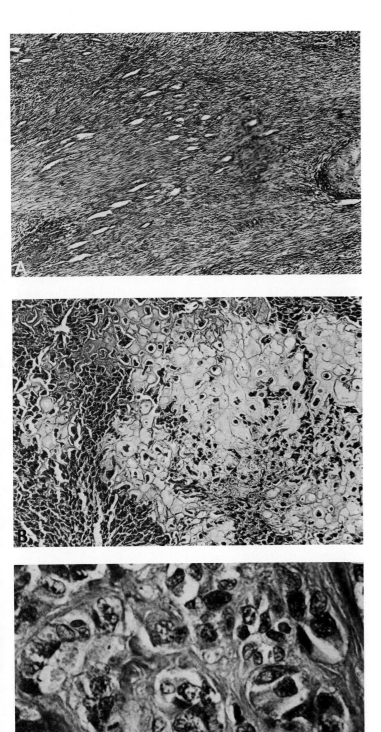

Fig. 11-4. Osteogenic sarcoma. *A*, Grade 1 fibroblastic. (Hematoxylin and eosin: x50.) *B*, Grade 3 chondroblastic. (Hematoxylin and eosin; x115.) *C*, Grade 4 osteoblastic. (Hematoxylin and eosin: x156.) (*B* from Dahlin DC: Bone Tumors: General Aspects and Data on 6,221 Cases. Third edition. Springfield, Illinois, Charles C Thomas, Publisher, 1978, p 241. By permission.)

Osteosarcoma and Its Variants

information is useful when planning the extent of the surgical procedure.

Staging of osteosarcoma is done primarily through examination of the lung fields. In the past, plain roentgenograms and tomograms were usually utilized to examine the lung fields. Currently, computed tomography (CT) is considered a much more sensitive and accurate way of ruling out pulmonary metastasis (5). In addition, CT of the lung fields is useful as a baseline against which subsequent studies can be measured during follow-up. In general, CT of the lung fields is better done before surgery is contemplated because the surgical procedure tends to produce small areas of atelectasis and fibrosis, which will be identified on CT and which may cause confusion.

Even before the biopsy procedure, the definitive procedure should be planned, if practical. Each case must be individualized and additional studies obtained as necessary. For example, if resection is being considered as an alternative to amputation, then it is helpful to know as precisely as possible the extent of the tumor and its relationship to the surrounding normal structures. CT of the primary lesion may be very helpful in this regard. Arteriography also may be helpful, particularly if major vessels are near the lesion. Sometimes arteriography can be combined with CT as a single procedure. Specialized situations may require additional examinations. For example, if the tumor arises in a pelvic bone, excretory urography may be done to determine the relationship of the tumor to the ureter and bladder. Again, the procedure can be combined with CT.

The Biopsy. Taking a biopsy specimen of a suspected bone tumor in a proper manner is critical, because improper placement of the biopsy incision may preclude surgical resection and necessitate an amputation. Transverse incisions on extremities are particularly troublesome and should be avoided. The biopsy incision must be placed so that it can be included in the resected specimen, if resection is indicated. The biopsy site also must be chosen to ensure that an adequate sample of representative tumor tissue can be delivered to the surgical pathologist. In general, the specimen should be obtained from the soft-tissue extension of the lesion, and the center of the lesion should not be cut. The tissue on the periphery is more accessible, easier to process in the pathology laboratory, and usually is the most malignant portion. Care must be taken, however, to avoid obtaining tissue from reactive new bone, which may be present at the junction between the periosteum and the soft-tissue extension of the tumor. Tissue from this area is benign. In general, incision of an overlying muscle to gain access to the tumor tissue is preferred over dissection between muscles, as one might do for a nontumorous condition. Meticulous hemostasis must be obtained, and the biopsy wound should be carefully closed. Many orthopedic oncologists believe that the biopsy procedure requires more skill and judgment than the surgical procedure.

Surgical Treatment. Although amputation is the treatment of choice for most osteosarcomas of the extremity, there is current interest in performing limb-salvage procedures as an alternative. This recent trend is probably due to two reasons: (1) the development of new surgical techniques and new methods of reconstruction and (2) enthusiasm for the use of pre-operative chemotherapy in an attempt to make tumors more readily resectable. A number of factors enter into the decision concerning the type of surgical procedure for a given patient: the age of the patient, stage of the disease, anatomic location of the tumor, size and degree of soft-tissue extension, and the histologic grade of the tumor.

Age. The age of the patient may influence the practicality of performing a resection as an alternative to amputation. For younger growing children, it is not practical to consider the insertion of metallic implants or customized total joints, except under most unusual circumstances. For these children, unless some alternative method of bone grafting is available, amputation probably is preferable. But older patients with limited life expectancy may benefit greatly from the use of a prosthetic device, whereas amputation might render them nonambulatory.

Stage of the Disease. Even in advanced disease, amputation is sometimes desirable as a palliative measure. For most patients who present with simultaneous primary and metastatic disease, an aggressive approach is indicated. If the patient is going to receive chemotherapy, this may influence the choice of reconstructive procedures available and may preclude the performance of some procedures. For example, bone grafting procedures, whether with autografts or allografts, probably should not be used if the patient is to receive cytotoxic chemotherapy.

Anatomic Location of the Tumor. Some tumors are so situated that they may be resected according to the principles of good tumor surgery without the need for extensive reconstructive procedures. For example, a lesion that involves the wing of the ilium may be simply resected, without the need for additional procedures. As another example, a tumor involving the fibula may be resected together with a cuff of surrounding normal tissue, with the expectation that there will be minimal functional deficit. Whenever the primary tumor is located in an expendable bone, surgical resection may be considered.

Size of the Lesion and Extent of Soft-Tissue Involvement. Whenever there is a very large tumor with considerable soft-tissue extension, amputation is probably the treatment of choice. However, if resection is considered, provision must be made for sacrifice of adjacent soft tissues. If these adjacent soft tissues are critical structures, such as major neurovascular structures, an important consideration is whether sacrifice of these structures will allow for the preservation of a functional and viable distal extremity. When there is a large tumor involving the bones in the region of the knee, with considerable soft-tissue extension, an alternative to amputation is the so-called Van Ness procedure or tibial turnaround procedure. This procedure entails essentially an intercalary amputation of the involved area with subsequent rotation of the remaining tibia through a 180° angle and reattachment of the distal limb in such a manner that the reversed ankle joint becomes a functional knee joint. A prosthesis can then be attached. With this procedure, the femoral artery can be sacrificed and subsequently reanastomosed. While this may seem a grotesque solution to a difficult surgical problem, the functional results may be amazingly good (6). In addition, patients treated in this manner have no problem with phantom limb sensations and seem to adjust psychologically at least as well as patients subjected to major amputations. In general, however, most orthopedic oncologists recommend amputation when the tumor is very large and has considerable soft-tissue extension. Alternatively, when a tumor is entirely confined to the bone with no soft-tissue extension, resection of the involved bone with a cuff of normal surrounding tissue may be considered.

Histologic Grade. In general, patients with high-grade osteosarcomas require amputation. This decision must always be balanced with the knowledge of the other factors involved. For example, even though the tumor may be high grade, if it is very small and entirely intraosseous, resection may be reasonably considered. Generally, most high-grade osteosarcomas tend to be fairly large at the outset, and patients with these tumors usually are not candidates for resection. The lower the grade of the tumor, the more reasonable it is to consider surgical resection as an alternative to amputation.

The Definitive Surgical Procedure

If, after consideration of all the foregoing factors, amputation is indicated, a decision must be made as to the level of amputation. This decision is particularly important when a tumor involves the distal femur. In this situation, one must consider whether to perform a high-thigh amputation, well above the most proximal extent of the tumor, or to perform a hip disarticulation. Some authorities advocate disarticulation because of the possibility of "skip" metastasis occurring within the medullary canal; however, such skip metastasis is relatively rarely encountered but, if present, is usually clinically apparent before the decision regarding the level of amputation has to be made. In other words, skip metastasis in the proximal femur is usually apparent on either the plain roentgenogram or the ^{99m}Tc bone scan before the decision has to be made regarding the level of amputation. My colleagues and I perform a cross-bone amputation through the proximal femur several inches below the lesser trochanter in an attempt to achieve a level of amputation of at least 8 cm above the most clinically apparent proximal level of extension of the tumor. Although the 8-cm rule is arbitrary, it has been effective—it allows for a margin of error.

During the past 15 years, we have had only two local recurrences in the proximal femur using this approach. Advocates of disarticulation have not demonstrated that the procedure improves the overall prognosis. If even a few centimeters of the proximal femur can be preserved, the functional results with a prosthesis are greatly improved as compared with the results when the entire femur is removed. Most orthopedic oncologists currently recommend cross-bone amputation rather than disarticulation, whenever this can be accomplished, with a reasonable margin of normal, uninvolved tissue.

When amputation is done, a cast pylon prosthesis should be applied immediately whenever possible; this not only allows for early functional recovery but also is very important for wound healing. Application of the cast pylon seems to aid in wound healing and control of local edema. The psychologic advantage of early ambulation is also important. Even with an upper extremity amputation, the early application of a cast prosthesis seems to be of definite benefit.

Most patients with newly diagnosed osteosarcomas are still best treated by primary amputation. With selected patients, however, the performance of so-called limb-salvage procedures seems warranted.

Surgical resection as an alternative to primary amputation may be considered because of a number of new developments in reconstructive surgery. For most primary bone tumors in the region of the knee which are amenable to resectional surgery, reconstruction is best accomplished by arthrodesis. If this can be accomplished, the result is a painless, stable knee; the obvious problem is lack of motion of the knee. Almost all the alternatives to arthrodesis are associated with instability or pain. For example, if the distal femur is resected and replaced with a custom-type total knee arthroplasty implant, there is considerable risk that the implant will fail through loosening, breakage, or wear. Alternatively, if an allograft is utilized, the allograft may not unite with the normal bone or osteoarthritis may develop subsequently in the joint. In either of these situations, a salvage procedure, which may require arthrodesis or even amputation, may be necessary.

A number of experimental approaches are currently being investigated in an effort to solve this problem. For example, a limb may be salvaged by the use of a large intercalary fibermetal implant, supplemented with autogenous iliac bone grafts utilized in such a manner as to achieve an arthrodesis of the knee (7). In the region of the hip joint, a tumor involving the proximal femur can be resected and the resected bone can be replaced with a custom-type total hip arthroplasty. However, little is currently known about the long-term results of such procedures. When a tumor of the diaphysis of a long bone is resected, several alternative methods of reconstruction are available. For example, an allograft might be utilized, with the expectation of a reasonably good result. Alternatively, a fibermetal implant might be utilized to bridge a large gap. Other innovative methods also have been tried. To date, there is no long-term information regarding the efficacy of any such trials, and all these methods of reconstruction should be considered experimental.

There is considerable need for input from the field of biomechanics. Numerous reconstructive procedures are now available. None of these procedures has been in use long enough to be definitely effective and reliable. Hence, considerably more information and discussion are needed before any definitive statements can be made regarding any one form of reconstructive surgery. For example, there have been reports of removal of the entire femur and replacement with a femoral prosthesis that has elements of both a total hip arthroplasty at one end and a total knee arthroplasty at the other end (8). While the initial reports of such a procedure may appear to be encouraging, the results of such treatment need to be observed for a prolonged period before any definitive statement may be made regarding the long-term efficacy of such treatment.

For most patients with classic high-grade osteosarcoma, amputation is the treatment of choice. Alternative approaches should be regarded as experimental. Long-term results of such experimental approaches may be efficacious, but such optimism is not currently warranted. Therefore, a patient with a large, high-grade lesion is probably best treated with amputation. With the development of more effective chemotherapy regimens, such patients may be treated by resection rather than amputation.

Adjunctive Treatment

Currently, considerable interest centers on adjunctive treatment after surgical removal of the primary tumor. There are a number of reasons why adjunctive treatment for osteosarcoma seems to be appropriate. The tumor tends to metastasize hematogenously and to spread to the peripheral lung fields. The lung fields are easily monitored by CT; hence, pulmonary metastatic lesions, in general, are rapidly detected. Therefore, it is relatively easy to determine the disease-free interval. When pulmonary metastatic lesions occur, they usually do so within the first 2 years after treatment of the primary lesion. Thus, the clinical results are obtained rapidly and the usefulness of a particular form of treatment can be determined. In addition, since most osteosarcomas occur in young people, there is the potential for long-term survival. From a theoretic standpoint, if the tumor burden can be reduced dramatically through either amputation or resection of the primary tumor, then the amount of tumor present in the body can be reduced to an extent that adjuvant chemotherapy can be expected to be effective. Numerous clinical trials have been done, with varying results (9). Most of these trials have reported significant improvement in survival as compared with the survival rate of 20% originally reported by Dahlin and Coventry (10) in 1967. The most recent trials note survival rates in excess of 50% at 5 years for patients treated by widely diverse adjunctive methods. The question is whether all of these diverse forms of treatment are effective in terms of achieving improved survival or whether there has been an improvement in survival because of some change in the natural history of osteosarcoma or in the method by which it is staged and treated (11).

The prognosis for current patients with osteosarcoma has improved over that for patients treated 20 years ago. When the initial report of Dahlin and Coventry was published in 1967, few believed the reported survival rate of 20%. Most investigators at that time believed that the rate noted by Dahlin and Coventry was too high. However, more critical analyses revealed that the 20% rate was approximately correct. In 1970, Marcove et al (12) published their results of the treatment of patients with osteosarcoma who were less than 21 years old and showed a 5-year survival rate of approximately 20%. Most subsequent investigators have tended to use this 20% rate as a standard against which their results may be compared. The acceptance of such a comparison was questioned by Rab et al (13) from the Mayo Clinic, in which patients were randomized to receive either surgery alone or surgery followed by so-called prophylactic radiation to both lung fields. There was no apparent improvement in survival for patients treated by radiation of the lung fields, but both groups of patients showed greatly improved survival as compared with historical controls. In another study from the Mayo Clinic (14) in which patients were randomized to receive a combination chemotherapy regimen containing methotrexate, doxorubicin, and vincristine or to receive transfer factor as immunotherapy, it was noted that there was no apparent advantage for either regimen. However, both regimens produced results that were much improved over those noted in historical controls.

The question, therefore, relates to whether all such forms of adjunctive treatment were effective or whether there was some improvement of survival that was independent of treatment. Subsequent analyses from the Mayo Clinic have shown a steadily improving survival—in terms of both disease-free interval and actual survival—in patients treated by surgery alone. These studies have questioned the results of adjunctive treatment programs which have claimed that the improvement in survival is due to the treatment. Currently, the subject remains controversial, and there is no general agreement as to whether any one particular form of adjunctive treatment is better than none at all (14).

However, a number of recent reports indicating greatly improved disease-free interval and actual survival merit attention. While most of these reports involve few patients followed for a short time, further follow-up may reveal worthwhile forms of adjunctive treatment (15). All are hopeful that these reports will be validated and proved to be efficacious. Without the use of concomitant untreated controls, however, it will be difficult to evaluate the value of such adjunctive treatment. The use of adjunctive chemotherapy remains theoretically desirable, and it is hoped by all concerned that such forms of treatment will prove to be of definite value.

Pulmonary Surgery

In the past, most thoracic surgeons believed that thoracic surgery for resection of a pulmonary lesion should be withheld unless the lesion remained solitary and showed little sign of progression over a period of observation. This usually meant that a patient with a pulmonary lesion would be observed for 3 to 6 months and thoracic surgery would be withheld unless there was little progression of the pulmonary disease. Martini et al (16) emphasized that osteosarcoma tends to metastasize to the periphery of the lung fields and that these lesions can be easily resected, with salvage of many patients. Since this approach has been utilized, many patients have been salvaged. Our current philosophy is that patients with pulmonary metastatic disease, in general, deserve exploration and resection of all apparent metastatic disease. The use of CT allows the early identification of such lesions and the more precise localization of the lesions. This approach has saved numerous patients who would otherwise have suffered progression and ultimately would have died of the disease. Approximately one-third of all patients with pulmonary metastasis may be "cured" by resection of pulmonary lesions (17). Whether or not the addition of so-called adjunctive chemotherapy after resection is of any value is currently debatable. In any case, all patients with osteosarcoma should be monitored closely for evidence of pulmonary metastasis, and if such metastasis occurs, prompt surgical intervention should be considered. It is important to realize that most such lesions occur in children and that these patients tolerate thoracic surgery amazingly well. Most children who undergo thoracotomy for resection of pulmonary disease are hospitalized approximately 5 days and may miss about a week of school. My colleagues and I do not hesitate to perform subsequent thoracotomies if they are indicated. Multiple thoracotomies seem to be tolerated reasonably well, with minimal loss of pulmonary function.

Follow-Up Examinations

Patients with osteosarcoma must be followed up closely and frequently for evidence of metastatic disease. Follow-up chest roentgenograms should be obtained at least every 6 weeks and tomographic examinations of the lung fields at least every 3 months during the first 2 years of observation. With this regimen, pulmonary metastasis may be detected early and the metastatic lesions may be resected at an early stage. CT of the lung fields is done as a preliminary staging procedure before any definitive surgical procedure is done; this study serves as a baseline against which follow-up studies may be compared. Any new lesions that are subsequently detected in young persons may be assumed to be metastatic disease. With this approach, we have had very few false-positive results of CT. Patients who are subjected to chemotherapeutic regimens may have their systemic immunity altered and may be subject to infectious diseases, with subsequent pulmonary scarring. For example, a patient who has received chemotherapy and who develops chickenpox may have chickenpox granulomas in the lung fields. Such lesions may cause confusion in the interpretation of the CT. In these rare situations, thoracic surgery may reveal the infectious nature of the problem and rule out the development of pulmonary metastatic disease.

Summary

Osteosarcoma is the most common primary sarcoma of bone. The lesion tends to occur in adolescents and young adults. A number of histologic variants of this lesion have been recognized. Classification of the disease is important for comparison of various clinical studies. Staging of the disease has improved considerably with the use of computed tomographic examination of the lung fields. Lesions which, in the past, were considered to be primary and localized may be metastatic from the onset. A number of new reconstructive procedures are now available which may allow for various limb-salvage procedures to be used as alternatives to amputation. Amputation remains the method of choice for most large high-grade osteosarcomas involving the extremities. Pulmonary resection for metastasis appears to be an extremely worthwhile procedure and should be considered whenever practical. A number of adjunctive chemotherapy regimens appear to be efficacious. However, the natural history of osteosarcoma may be changing in that patients treated by surgery alone appear to have improved disease-free intervals and actual survival. The exact value of adjunctive treatment remains to be proved. It is hoped that one or more such chemotherapeutic regimens will be of established value.

References
1. Lichtenstein L: Bone Tumors. Fourth edition. St Louis, CV Mosby Company, 1972, p 224
2. Dahlin DC, Unni KK: Osteosarcoma of bone and its important recognizable varieties. Am J Surg Pathol 1:61–72, 1977
3. Enneking WF, Kagan A: "Skip" metastases in osteosarcoma. Cancer 36:2192–2205, 1975
4. Dahlin DC: Bone Tumors: General Aspects and Data on 6,221 Cases. Third edition. Springfield, Illinois, Charles C Thomas, Publisher, 1978, p 239
5. Muhm JR, Pritchard DJ: Computer tomography for the detection of

pulmonary metastasis in patients with osteogenic sarcoma (abstract). Proc Am Assoc Cancer Res 21:148, 1980

6. Salzer M, Knahr K, Kotz R, et al: Treatment of osteosarcomata of the distal femur by rotation-plasty. Arch Orthop Trauma Surg 99:131–136, 1981

7. Andersson GBJ, Gaechter A, Galante JO, et al: Segmental replacement of long bones in baboons using a fiber titanium implant. J Bone Joint Surg [Am] 60:31–40, 1978

8. Rosen G, Murphy ML, Huvos AG, et al: Chemotherapy, *en bloc* resection, and prosthetic bone replacement in the treatment of osteogenic sarcoma. Cancer 37:1–11, 1976

9. Benjamin RS: Adjuvant chemotherapy for osteosarcoma. *In* Controversies in Oncology. Edited by P Wiernik. New York, John Wiley & Sons, 1982, pp 125–187

10. Dahlin DC, Coventry MB: Osteogenic sarcoma: a study of six hundred cases. J Bone Joint Surg [Am] 49:101–110, 1967

11. Taylor WF, Ivins JC, Dahlin DC, et al: Trends and variability in survival from osteosarcoma. Mayo Clin Proc 53:695–700, 1978

12. Marcove RC, Miké V, Hajek JV, et al: Osteogenic sarcoma under the age of twenty-one: a review of one hundred and forty-five operative cases. J Bone Joint Surg [Am] 52:411–423, 1970

13. Rab GT, Ivins JC, Childs DS Jr, et al: Elective whole lung irradiation in the treatment of osteogenic sarcoma. Cancer 38:939–942, 1976

14. Pritchard DJ: Is adjuvant chemotherapy of osteosarcoma of proved value? *In* Controversies in Oncology. Edited by P Wiernik. New York, John Wiley & Sons, 1982, pp 189–194

15. Rosen G, Marcove RC, Caparros B, et al: Primary osteogenic sarcoma: the rationale for preoperative chemotherapy and delayed surgery. Cancer 43:2163–2177, 1979

16. Martini N, Huvos AG, Miké V, et al: Multiple pulmonary resections in the treatment of osteogenic sarcoma. Ann Thorac Surg 12:271–278, 1971

17. Telander RL, Pairolero PC, Pritchard DJ, et al: Resection of pulmonary metastatic osteogenic sarcoma in children. Surgery 84:335–340, 1978

CHAPTER 12

CHONDROSARCOMA AND ITS VARIANTS

Thomas C. Shives, M.D.
Lester E. Wold, M.D.
David C. Dahlin, M.D.
John W. Beabout, M.D.

Chondrosarcoma is a challenging neoplasm because its true nature is not widely appreciated, particularly as regards the histologic evaluation and degree of malignancy. Chondrosarcoma is a malignant tumor whose cells produce hyaline cartilage that is usually lobulated (1). Most chondrosarcomas are either well differentiated or moderately well differentiated, coinciding with an often prolonged clinical evolution (months or years). The cytologic features, however, of the common well-differentiated sarcoma are only subtly different from those of benign neoplasms of hyaline cartilage, and the pathologist must often rely on clinical data or radiographic features to aid in diagnosis.

In addition to the problems experienced by the pathologist in diagnosing this lesion, chondrosarcoma is therapeutically challenging and unfortunately may be easily mismanaged. Because chondrosarcoma frequently occurs in the proximal limbs or pelvis, surgical treatment may be difficult or impossible. This problem may be compounded by late diagnosis because of the insidious onset and late progession of symptoms due to slow growth of the lesion. Finally, the imperfect knowledge of the biologic potential of this lesion, particularly its propensity for local recurrence, may lead to treatment that is not radical enough (2). In addition to "primary" chondrosarcomas that arise in previously normal bone, those that develop as a result of the malignant degeneration of benign cartilaginous tumors are referred to as "secondary" chondrosarcomas. The original lesion is most commonly an osteochondroma (especially in patients with multiple, familial osteochondromatosis) and is less often a chondroma (enchondroma) (3).

A chondrosarcoma also can be classified as "peripheral" or "central," depending on its position in the affected bone. A chondrosarcoma that develops within the interior of a bone may be designated a central chondrosarcoma and one that begins in the cartilaginous cap of an osteochondroma, a peripheral chondrosarcoma.

There are several "variants" of chondrosarcoma which should be recognized because of their distinctive histologic appearances and different biologic behaviors.

Ordinary Chondrosarcoma

Chondrosarcoma is basically a lesion of middle-aged and older adults. Most tumors tend to occur in patients who are in the third to seventh decades (2,3). Most cases in the Mayo Clinic files involved patients who were in the fifth and sixth decades (3) (Fig. 12-1). "Secondary" chondrosarcomas tend to occur in patients who are approximately 10 years younger (3,4).

In most large series, the majority of chondrosarcomas involve the long bones (especially the femur) and bones of the pelvis (2–5). When a long bone is affected, the lesion most often originates near the end of the diaphysis or metaphysis. Lesions are rarely found in the central portion of the diaphysis. It is

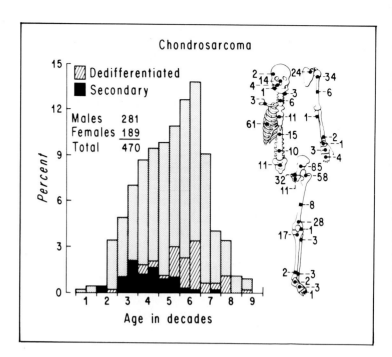

Fig. 12-1. Age, sex, and site distribution of chondrosarcomas seen at Mayo Clinic up to Jan. 1, 1979. (From Dahlin DC: Bone Tumors: General Aspects and Data on 6,221 Cases. Third edition. Springfield, Illinois, Charles C Thomas, Publisher, 1978. By permission.)

noteworthy that chondrosarcoma below the level of the wrist and ankle is distinctly rare. Lesions of the pelvis most commonly affect the acetabular region.

Symptoms are generally mild and insidious in onset. A long clinical evolution is characteristic. Local swelling or pain (or both) is usually the presenting symptom. The presence of a mass usually makes the diagnosis easier, but in many cases, especially in tumors arising in the innominate bone, reliance must be placed on the radiographic appearance for diagnosis. The presence of pain is reliable evidence of active growth in a central cartilage lesion (3). Patients with peripheral chondrosarcoma often have exostoses that continue to enlarge (2).

The radiograph usually provides important information in the diagnosis of chondrosarcoma, and the findings often are pathognomonic. These tumors usually are seen as an area of bone destruction in the medullary portion of the bone. Typically, the margins of the tumor are poorly defined. Mineralization of the tumor matrix is common and presents as a characteristic type of calcification, often referred to as punctate, flocculent, or ring-like (Fig. 12-2).

The indolent nature of chondrosarcoma usually becomes apparent when the bone has an increased diameter and a thickened cortex (Fig. 12-3). Rarely, chondrosarcomas are purely osteolytic.

In central cartilage tumors, the presence of endosteal erosion or destruction is an important sign of malignancy, and this gives a scalloped appearance to the endosteum. Tumors with this

214

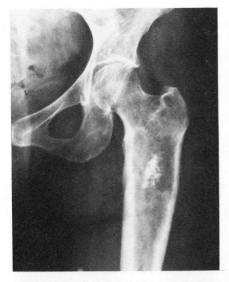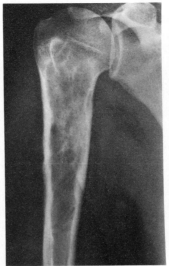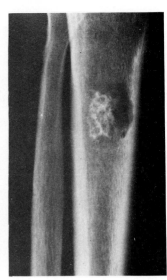

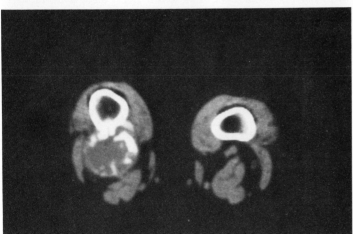

Fig. 12-5.

Fig. 12-2. Chondrosarcoma with typical cartilaginous calcification.

Fig. 12-3. Chondrosarcoma with widened medullary canal plus thickened cortex. Changes similar to those seen in Figure 12-2, except there is no calcification.

Fig. 12-4. Central low-grade chondrosarcoma with endosteal destruction of cortex. There is also a lytic area in the central lesion.

Fig. 12-5. CT scan indicating soft-tissue extension of chondrosarcoma in posterior aspect of thigh. Medullary canal is normal.

pattern are usually of lower grade malignancy and are often considered "borderline" malignant by pathologists (Fig. 12-4).

Computed tomography is helpful in evaluating cartilage tumors, particularly those located in the trunk. It allows accurate delineation of the tumor, including any soft-tissue extension (Fig. 12-5).

A secondary chondrosarcoma arising in an osteochondroma is usually readily apparent radiographically. The findings, suggestive of malignant transformation, are the presence of a soft-tissue mass or destruction within the ossified portion of the exostosis or both a mass and destruction (Fig. 12-6).

Grossly, chondrosarcomas are usually lobulated, with lobules being less distinct at the periphery of the tumor, where they tend to coalesce. The tumors vary in consistency from firm to

Chondrosarcoma and Its Variants

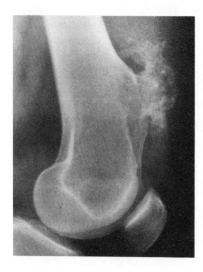

Fig. 12-6. Secondary chondrosarcoma arising in typical osteochondroma. There is bone destruction in periphery of osteochondroma plus a soft-tissue mass.

Fig. 12-7. Chondrosarcoma. This chondrosarcoma has characteristic chondroid islands in femoral neck and extending into proximal diaphysis. Tumor is entirely intramedullary, and no foci of dedifferentiation are noted.

soft and myxoid and have a semitranslucent white to gray color. Yellow foci of calcification occasionally may be identified. A myxoid quality to the tumor is strongly suggestive that the lesion is malignant. The myxoid quality of these tumors may result in cyst formation, which can be appreciated on gross inspection (Fig. 12-7).

Microscopically, chondrosarcoma presents an extremely varied pattern. The findings range from patterns that are difficult to distinguish from those of chondromas to patterns that are high-grade and poorly differentiated. Although the cellularity of cartilage tumors overall correlates poorly with prognosis (chondromas of the hands and feet may be cellular and still behave in a benign fashion), this feature is helpful when differentiating benign chondroid tumor from sarcoma of the trunk. Nuclear anaplasia is another important indicator of malignancy. Finally, the presence of numerous binucleated cells correlates with the malignant potential. Even given these criteria, differentiating the low-grade chondrosarcoma from the cellular-active chondroma may be extremely difficult (Fig. 12-8 and 12-9).

In order to evaluate the cartilaginous tumor suspected of being malignant, an incisional biopsy is recommended. The incision should be planned and performed so that definitive treatment will include removal of the biopsy wound in its entirety, along with the tumor. This approach minimizes the chance of seeding and local recurrence.

In addition, a significant tumor volume may be needed for

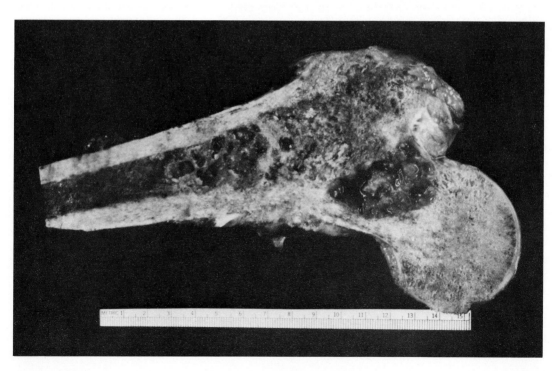

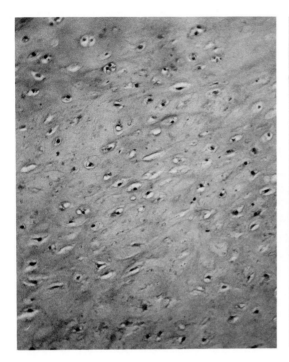 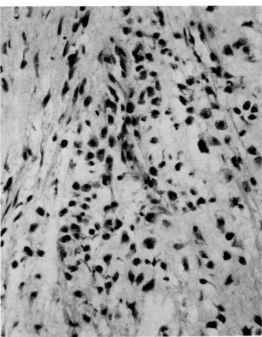

pathologic examination because the diagnosis must be based on viable and unaltered zones of neoplastic tissue and not on areas that have undergone necrosis (2).

Treatment of chondrosarcoma is surgical. The literature is replete with statements discounting any beneficial effect of radiation therapy (2,4, 6,7). At the present time, there appears to be no definite role for adjunctive chemotherapy.

Adequate treatment of chondrosarcoma requires surgical ablation, with the goals being those for any malignant bone tumor, that is, eradication of the lesion and preservation of as much function as possible. However, the subsequent development of recurrences in many surgically treated patients attests to the fact that surgery is often inadequate (1). The lesion is usually controlled best by adequate en bloc resection or amputation. Obviously, amputation accomplishes the most complete ablation and therefore gives the best chance of long-term survival. However, if a limb-sparing procedure can be accomplished and if the entire tumor can be resected, the possibility of long-term survival is not altered (8). Of paramount importance in planning adequate surgery is a careful preoperative assessment. Use of computed tomography is particularly valuable in the preoperative assessment of both the intraosseous and the extraosseous extent of the lesion.

Generally, chondrosarcoma is believed to be less malignant than osteogenic sarcoma. However, this inherent "advantage" for chondrosarcoma may be offset by difficulties, delays, and

Fig. 12-8. Chondrosarcoma. Well-differentiated (grade 1) chondrosarcoma may mimic histologic appearance of enchondromas, as in this case. Binucleated cells or cells with hyperchromatic nuclei may be inconspicuous. A radiographically malignant appearance is necessary collaborative evidence to designate such a lesion as a grade 1 chondrosarcoma. (Hematoxylin and eosin; x160.)

Fig. 12-9. Chondrosarcoma. Poorly differentiated (high-grade) chondrosarcoma shows cytologic features of malignancy, that is, anaplasia, hyperchromatism, and so forth. The chondroid nature of the tumor may not be obvious in a given microscopic field. (Hematoxylin and eosin; x400.)

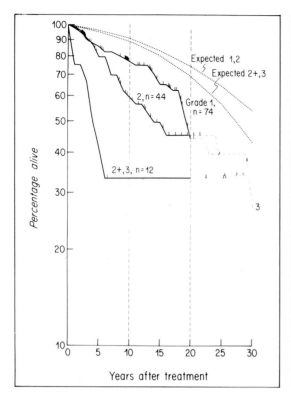

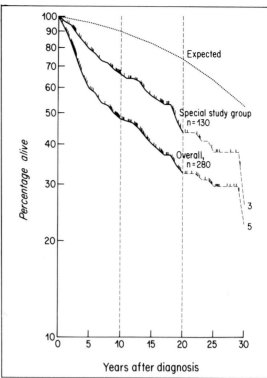

Fig. 12-10. Survival according to histologic grade in a group of 130 patients who underwent curative-type surgery at the Mayo Clinic between 1909 and 1975. (From Pritchard DJ, Lunke RJ, Taylor WF, et al: Chondrosarcoma: a clinicopathologic and statistical analysis. Cancer 45:149–157, 1980. By permission of the American Cancer Society.)

Fig. 12-11. Overall survival of 280 patients who were treated at the Mayo Clinic between 1909 and 1975. The special study group includes patients who underwent curative surgery at the Mayo Clinic. (From Pritchard DJ, Lunke RJ, Taylor WF, et al: Chondrosarcoma: a clinicopathologic and statistical analysis. Cancer 45:149–157, 1980. By permission of the American Cancer Society.)

mistakes in diagnosis and treatment (2). Although the histologic interpretation of these tumors is often extremely difficult, a definite correlation exists between histologic grade of the tumor and overall survival. Patients with low-grade lesions have a distinctly improved disease-free interval and overall survival than do patients with higher grade lesions (Fig. 12-10). Overall, the 5-year survival rate is approximately 50% (2,8) (Fig. 12-11). Patients with central lesions (trunk and pelvis) have a poorer prognosis than do patients with lesions located in the limbs. In addition to the histologic grade, the size of the lesion appears to be the other most significant prognostic factor (Fig. 12-12). Control of the primary lesion is of critical importance. Local recurrence adversely affects survival (8).

For the future, a greater understanding of the histologic features of this disease should result in a more prompt, accurate diagnosis. Likewise, better knowledge of the behavior of this tumor and the avoidance of potential pitfalls in the surgical management should improve the overall prognosis.

Mesenchymal Chondrosarcoma

Although mesenchymal chondrosarcoma is of relatively recent delineation, it is now well recognized because of its distinctive histologic pattern and unusual clinical features (9). Nearly

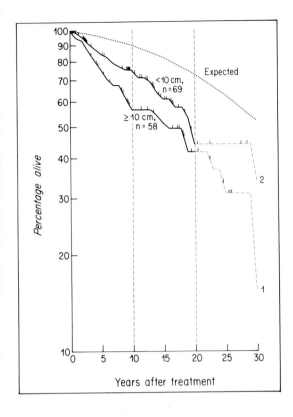

Fig. 12-12. Survival according to tumor size in 127 patients treated at the Mayo Clinic.

one-third of the cases reported in the literature have involved lesions of soft-tissue origin (10). Most patients were in the second and third decades of life, with a slight preponderance of females (10). The tumors have been found in many skeletal sites, but in contrast to most tumors of bone, mesenchymal chondrosarcomas rarely involve the tubular bones (Fig. 12-13).

The usual presenting symptom of pain or a mass (or both) is of little diagnostic value.

Roentgenographically, mesenchymal chondrosarcomas arising in bone are primarily osteolytic. The margins may be fairly sharply defined, but usually they fade gradually and imperceptibly into the surrounding normal bone. Most lesions have calcific deposits in an overall pattern that is usually indistinguishable from the pattern of ordinary chondrosarcoma.

Grossly, the tumor is usually soft gray-white or yellow, with firm cartilaginous areas intermixed (10). A bimorphic pattern is confirmed on microscopic study. The gray-white areas are composed of small round or oval cells that often are arranged in a hemangiopericytoid fashion. Almost benign-appearing chondroid islands are admixed in this small-cell malignant background, giving the tumor its characteristic histologic pattern. (Fig. 12-14).

Although the clinical courses in the reported cases have been variable and often prolonged, the biologic behavior of mesen-

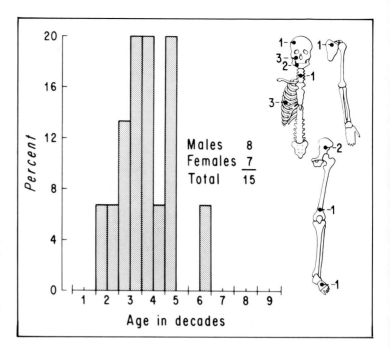

Fig. 12-13. Age, sex, and site distribution of mesenchymal chondrosarcomas seen at the Mayo Clinic up to Jan. 1, 1979. (From Dahlin DC: Bone Tumors: General Aspects and Data on 6,221 Cases. Third edition. Springfield, Illinois, Charles C Thomas, Publisher, 1978. By permission.)

chymal chondrosarcoma is usually relentless, with a strong capacity for producing metastasis (9–11). Patients with this lesion probably are best treated by radical surgery to achieve complete ablation.

Dedifferentiated Chondrosarcoma

Of all the recognized variants of chondrosarcoma, the dedifferentiated chondrosarcoma is of special importance because of its highly malignant nature and correspondingly poor prognosis. Dahlin and Beabout (12) define this category of tumors as having contiguity of histologic grade 1 (or "borderline") chondrosarcomatous areas with juxtaposed zones of anaplastic fibrosarcoma or osteogenic sarcoma. Others (13) have reported different forms of sarcoma associated with a low-grade cartilaginous lesion. Dedifferentiation occurs in about 10% of chondrosarcomas (3). The cartilaginous component may be either a primary or a recurrent low-grade chondrosarcoma. The patient age distribution and the skeletal location in dedifferentiated chondrosarcomas are similar to those in ordinary chondrosarcoma. The most frequent site of the tumors in the Mayo Clinic files was the innominate bone (Fig. 12-15), whereas the femur was the most frequent site in Campanacci and associates' series (13). The symptoms of pain and swelling are likewise similar to those seen with any bone tumor, although the duration of symptoms is usually longer than would be anticipated on the basis of the dedifferentiated, anaplastic portions of the tumor.

Radiographically, these tumors are usually large. A portion

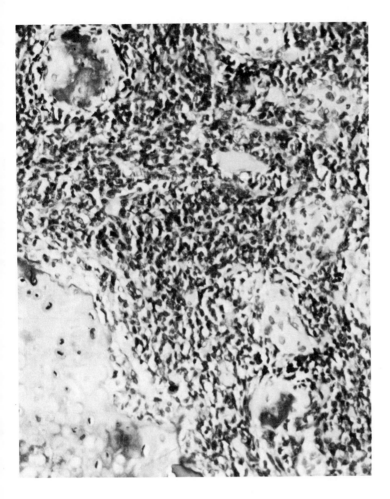

Fig. 12-14. Mesenchymal chondrosarcoma. Bimorphic pattern of mesenchymal chondrosarcoma is illustrated. Hemangiopericytoid areas alternate with chondroid islands. (Hematoxylin and eosin; x250.)

of the lesion will have the characteristic appearance of a low-grade chondrosarcoma, and adjacent to it will be an area that appears to be more aggressive than would be expected in a chondrosarcoma. Destruction of the cortex is seen in the dedifferentiated area, and an associated soft-tissue mass is usually present (Fig. 12-16).

Grossly, the tumor often has a central cartilaginous, semitranslucent bluish white region. The lobulation and calcification of low-grade chondrosarcoma are evident in these regions. In some tumors, this portion may be so small as to be overlooked. The low-grade portions of the tumor abut upon grayer, softer, more friable anaplastic portions (Fig. 12-17). The microscopic appearance of the tumor confirms the gross features. There are abrupt transitions from low-grade chondrosarcoma to anaplastic osteosarcoma or fibrosarcoma. Sometimes the highly malignant portions show the pattern of malignant fibrous histiocytoma. The intimate admixture and abrupt transition are features that facilitate the separation of dedifferentiated chondrosarcoma from chondroblastic osteosarcoma (Fig. 12-18).

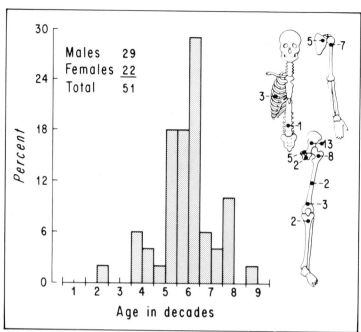

Fig. 12-15

Fig. 12-15. Age, sex, and site distribution of dedifferentiated chondrosarcomas seen at Mayo Clinic up to Jan. 1, 1979. (From Dahlin DC: Bone Tumors: General Aspects and Data on 6,221 Cases. Third edition. Springfield, Illinois, Charles C Thomas, Publisher, 1978. By permission.)

Fig. 12-16. Typical cartilaginous calcification in condylar portion of femur. Proximal to this, there is lytic, permeative destruction of cortex, indicating a highly aggressive lesion. This combination of findings is suggestive of dedifferentiation.

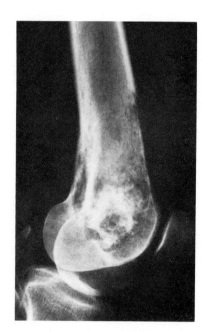

Currently, the differential diagnosis is of more than academic interest because of the various therapeutic modalities that are being used in the treatment of osteosarcoma.

Dedifferentiated chondrosarcomas represent one of the most malignant neoplasms of bone, and the prognosis is unfavorable. In the series reported by Dahlin and Beabout (12), 23 of 28 patients with follow-up of 2 years or longer died of their disease. Treatment, therefore, must be radical and dictated by the dedifferentiated portion of the tumor. The implication of the possibility of dedifferentiation is important to consider in the treatment of a cartilaginous tumor. Although small, this risk emphasizes the need for adequate, often aggressive, treatment of a primary cartilage malignant lesion, so that the threat of recurrence is minimized. Dedifferentiation also may account for the development of a rapidly growing recurrence in a previously treated chondrosarcoma.

Clear Cell Chondrosarcoma

Clear cell chondrosarcomas constitute a very small group of lesions which, before their description by Unni and others in 1976 (14), had frequently been mistaken for chondroblastomas or osteoblastomas. Of low-grade malignancy, these chondrosarcomas were so named because of their peculiar histologic appearance.

All affected patients have been adults, with an age range from 18 to 68 years (14–16). Nearly all lesions have been located in the epiphysis or metaphysis of a long bone. Symptoms are

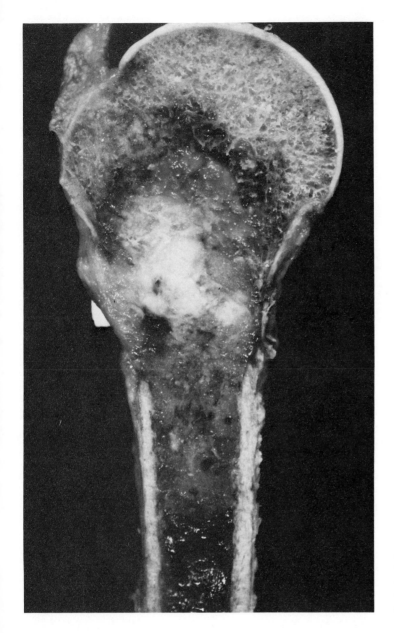

Fig. 12-17. Dedifferentiated chondrosarcoma. In addition to chondroid islands, this tumor from proximal humerus shows a central sclerotic zone. Such foci are characteristic of dedifferentiation in chondrosarcomas.

generally of long duration and are frequently referable to the adjacent joint. Pathologic fractures are not uncommon.

The roentgenographic appearance is usually not diagnostic. Typically, osteolytic expansion at the end of a long bone is seen. The cortex generally remains intact but is frequently expanded. The margins of the lesion are usually well defined, except in larger lesions, where the borders may be indistinct. Evidence of calcification within the lesion is uncommon (Fig. 12-19).

Chondrosarcoma and Its Variants

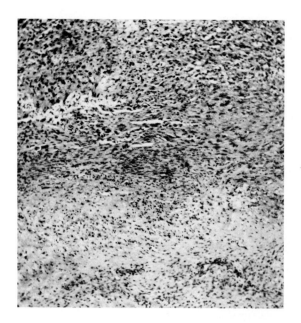

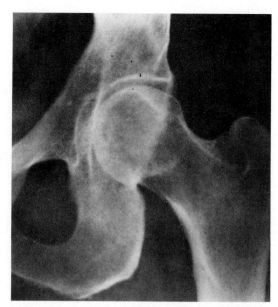

Fig. 12-18. Dedifferentiated chondrosarcoma. Anaplastic, high-grade areas within these tumors may have the histologic appearance of osteosarcoma, fibrosarcoma, or even malignant fibrous histiocytoma. Areas of low-grade chondrosarcoma are scattered within these anaplastic zones. (Hematoxylin and eosin; x100.)

Fig. 12-19. Clear cell chondrosarcoma. Lesion is purely lytic and near the end of the bone. In some areas, the margins are well defined. Margin is poorly defined distally.

Microscopically, the tumor is composed of cells with abundant clear cytoplasm and distinct cell boundaries. Intimately admixed with these cells are numerous benign multinucleated giant cells occurring singly or in small clusters (Fig. 12-20). Because of its confusion with benign lesions, clear cell chondrosarcoma has generally been treated too conservatively. The lesion is capable of metastasizing. Complete total resection is the treatment of choice.

References

1. Henderson ED, Dahlin DC: Chondrosarcoma of bone: a study of two hundred and eighty-eight cases. J Bone Joint Surg [Am] 45:1450–1458, 1963
2. Campanacci M, Guernelli N, Leonessa C, et al: Chondrosarcoma: a study of 133 cases, 80 with long term follow up. Ital J Orthop Traumatol 1:387–414, 1975
3. Dahlin DC: Bone Tumors: General Aspects and Data on 6,221 Cases. Third edition. Springfield, Illinois, Charles C Thomas, Publisher, 1978
4. Lindbom, A, Söderberg G, Spjut HJ: Primary chondrosarcoma of bone. Acta Radiol (Stockh) 55:81–96, 1961
5. O'Neal LW, Ackerman LV: Chondrosarcoma of bone. Cancer 5:551–577, 1952
6. Platt H: Survival in bone sarcoma. Acta Orthop Scand 32:267–280, 1962
7. McKenna RJ, Schwinn CP, Soong KY, et al: Sarcomata of the osteogenic series (osteosarcoma, fibrosarcoma, chondrosarcoma, parosteal osteogenic sarcoma, and sarcomata arising in abnormal bone): an analysis of 552 cases. J Bone Joint Surg [Am] 48:1–26, 1966
8. Pritchard DJ, Lunke RJ, Taylor WF, et al: Chondrosarcoma: a clinicopathologic and statistical analysis. Cancer 45:149–157, 1980

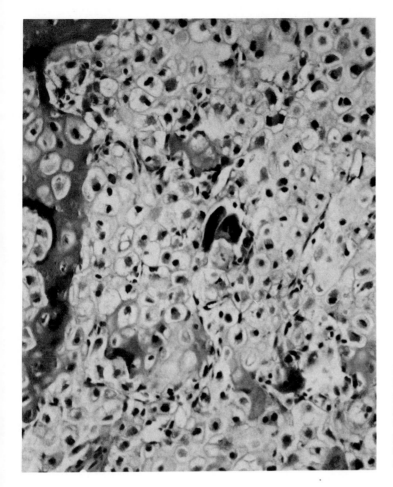

Fig. 12-20. Clear cell chondrosarcoma. Histologically, these tumors are composed of cells with abundant clear cytoplasm. Giant cells scattered throughout the tumor may result in a histologic appearance similar to that of osteoblastoma or chondroblastoma. (Hematoxylin and eosin; x250.)

9. Lichtenstein L, Bernstein D: Unusual benign and malignant chondroid tumors of bone: a survey of some mesenchymal cartilage tumors and malignant chondroblastic tumors, including a few multicentric ones, as well as many atypical benign chondroblastomas and chondromyxoid fibromas. Cancer 12:1142–1157, 1959
10. Salvador AH, Beabout JW, Dahlin DC: Mesenchymal chondrosarcoma: observations on 30 new cases. Cancer 28:605–615, 1971
11. Goldman RL: "Mesenchymal" chondrosarcoma, a rare malignant chondroid tumor usually primary in bone: report of a case arising in extraskeletal soft tissue. Cancer 20:1494–1498, 1967
12. Dahlin DC, Beabout JW: Dedifferentiation of low-grade chondrosarcomas. Cancer 28:461–466, 1971
13. Campanacci M, Bertoni F, Capanna R: Dedifferentiated chondrosarcomas. Ital J Orthop Traumatol 5:331–341, 1979
14. Unni KK, Dahlin DC, Beabout JW, et al: Chondrosarcoma: clear-cell variant; report of sixteen cases. J Bone Joint Surg [Am] 58:676–683, 1976
15. Campanacci M, Bertoni F, Laus M: Clear cell chondrosarcoma. Ital J Orthop Traumatol 6:365–372, 1980
16. Le Charpentier Y, Forest M, Postel M, et al: Clear-cell chondrosarcoma: a report of five cases including ultrastructural study. Cancer 44:622–629, 1979

CHAPTER 13

FIBROSARCOMA

Franklin H. Sim, M.D.
Lester E. Wold, M.D.
Krishnan K. Unni, M.B., B.S.
Richard A. McLeod, M.D.

Fibrosarcoma of bone is recognized as a distinctive clinical and pathologic entity characterized by fibroblastic malignant cells that do not produce osteoid (1–3). MacDonald and Budd (4) and later Phemister (5) were among the first to support the concept of fibrosarcoma of bone as a distinctive primary bone neoplasm. Others denied its existence, indicating that it represents an undifferentiated osteogenic sarcoma or invasion of bone secondarily from a soft-tissue fibrosarcoma (3). However, there is now ample clinical, pathologic, and experimental evidence to resolve this controversy (6–9). Generally, this primary malignant neoplasm arises from the supporting connective tissue elements of the medullary or cortical regions (central), although some of the lesions begin in the periosteum (periosteal).

Fibrosarcoma is a relatively rare osseous lesion. The files of the Mayo Clinic to Jan. 1, 1976, include 158 cases of primary fibrosarcoma of bone, which is less than 4% of the primary malignant bone tumors in the series. Osteogenic sarcoma was diagnosed in 962 cases. If a predominantly fibroblastic tumor produced even a small focus of osteoid, we considered it a fibroblastic osteosarcoma.

Clinical Features

Clinically, patients with fibrosarcoma of bone may be of any age, but generally they are adults of middle age. In our series, only one patient, a 6-year-old girl, was less than 10 years of age. The ages ranged from 6 to 86 years, with 24% of the patients in the fourth decade of life. This age distribution is in accord with that found by other observers (2,6) and contrasts with the peak incidence of osteogenic sarcoma in the second decade of life. Although some observers have noted a slight preponderance of female patients (10), there was no sex predilection in the Mayo Clinic series (Fig. 13-1).

The symptoms and signs of fibrosarcoma of bone are not specific, and like other osseous neoplasms, fibrosarcomas frequently have an insidious onset, which does not promote early recognition. There is usually a long delay before diagnosis. The presenting clinical complaints in the Mayo Clinic series (1), as in most series of bone tumors, were pain and swelling and varied considerably in duration, being present for more than 1 year in 18 cases and more than 2 years in 4 of 114 cases reported from our institution in 1969 (11). In Gilmer and MacEwen's series (10), the average duration of symptoms before diagnosis was 8 months, and other authors also have reported a long duration of symptoms before diagnosis (2). The physical findings vary, depending on the location and the extent of the lesion. Local tenderness with or without a palpable mass is most frequently present, and occasionally there is local heat and restriction of motion in the involved region. A pathologic fracture through the region of fibrosarcoma occasionally may be the initial complaint (Fig. 13-2).

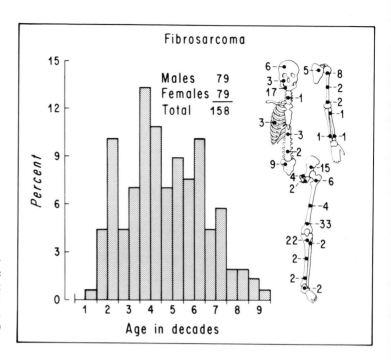

Fig. 13-1. Age and sex distribution of patients with fibrosarcoma in the Mayo Clinic Series. (From Dahlin DC: Bone Tumors: General Aspects and Data on 6,221 Cases. Third edition. Springfield, Illinois, Charles C Thomas, Publishers, 1978, p 316. By permission.)

The femur and the tibia are the sites most frequently affected, accounting for 43.6% in the Mayo Clinic series (Fig. 13-1). This distribution parallels the observations of other authors and does not differ from the distribution for osteogenic sarcoma (2,6,10). Similarly, the tumor usually is metaphyseal, 36% occurring near the knee. In addition, 26 patients in the Mayo Clinic series had primary fibrosarcoma involving the skull and jaws, 21 the pelvis, 15 the spinal column and sacrum, 3 the ribs, and 2 the calcaneus.

The lesion usually is solitary, but in certain rare cases, multiple independent tumors may develop simultaneously over the entire skeleton (12,13). This was the clinical presentation in one patient in the Mayo Clinic series. Fibrosarcoma may arise in bones affected by preexisting disease. Several predisposing causes for the development of secondary fibrosarcoma of bone have been reported (14,15). Of the 158 lesions in the Mayo Clinic series, 43 involved contributing causes, and the fibrosarcomas were regarded as "secondary lesions." Twenty-nine of these "secondary" fibrosarcomas occurred after radiation therapy.

Malignant change in a giant cell tumor of bone, usually with previous therapeutic radiation, may present as a fibrosarcoma. Similarly, fibrosarcoma may develop as an untoward sequel to irradiation of other types of diseased bone, as well as in normal bone in the field of irradiation. Of 70 patients with postirradiation sarcomas who were seen at the Mayo Clinic, 29 had fibrosarcomas. Secondary fibrosarcoma has been reported in preexisting Paget's disease of bone. Only 5 of the 158 lesions were associated with Paget's disease. Less commonly, secondary

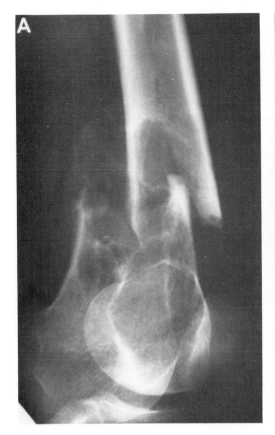 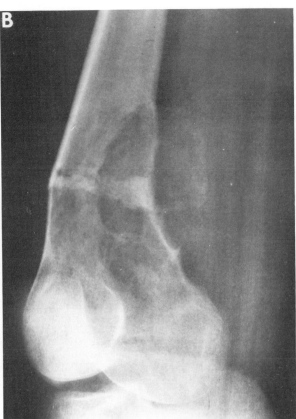

fibrosarcoma of bone may arise in areas of long-standing osteomyelitis and rarely in association with fibrous dysplasia of bone.

Fig. 13-2. Oblique (*A*) and lateral (*B*) views of distal femur showing malignant destructive lesion with a pathologic fracture. There is cortical destruction and soft-tissue extension. Biopsy revealed a malignant fibrohistiocytoma. The patient underwent high thigh amputation.

Roentgenographic Features

Radiologically, fibrosarcoma is an osteolytic lesion, and although the roentgenographic findings are not pathognomonic, the characteristic destructiveness usually gives conclusive evidence of the malignant nature of the lesion (Fig. 13-3). Permeative growth often gives a mottled radiolucency. With cortical destruction, extension into soft tissues commonly occurs. Periosteal bone reaction may be seen. There are no roentgenographic features that distinguish fibrosarcoma from osteolytic osteogenic sarcoma, and the roentgenographic appearance is often difficult to distinguish from that of solitary metastasis, myeloma, lymphoma, or rarely benign "cystic" lesions of bone.

Pathologic Findings

Pathologically, the tumor has a distinctive growth pattern. It may be composed of a firm fibrous mass of tissue or of soft

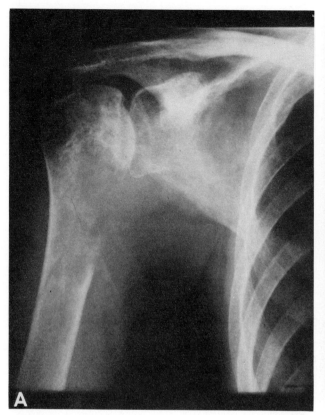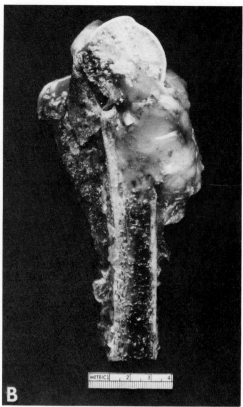

Fig. 13-3. *A*, Anteroposterior view of left shoulder showing lytic destruction of proximal humerus. Cortex is destroyed and there is soft-tissue extension. *B*, Gross specimen after forequarter amputation.

fleshy tissue, sometimes even myxoid, that invades the bone irregularly. Pseudoencapsulation may occur. Usually, cortical destruction and breakthrough are evident, with a variable amount of soft-tissue extension. Metastasis is usually hematogenous and occurs most commonly to the lungs.

Fibrosarcoma in bone has the same histologic pattern as that of fibrosarcoma of soft tissue (Fig. 13-4), except that the former invades and destroys bone. The cytologic appearance varies greatly. The degree of differentiation of the malignant fibroblasts, the histologic pattern, and the amount of collagen produced are also variable. The well-differentiated tumor may be difficult to differentiate from a desmoplastic fibroma or fibrous dysplasia. The poorly differentiated or high-grade tumors are anaplastic neoplasms that must be differentiated from malignant fibrous histiocytoma and metastatic "spindling" carcinoma.

The fibrosarcomas in the Mayo Clinic series were graded on the basis of cytologic features by the Broders method; most were moderately well or poorly differentiated, only a few being well differentiated. In a report of 114 cases (11), 30 lesions were classified as grade 4, 48 as grade 3, 35 as grade 2, and only 1 as grade 1.

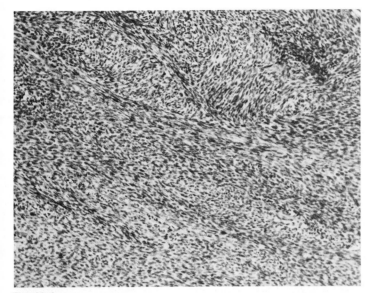

Fig. 13-4.

Fig. 13-4. Fibrosarcoma in bone shows same histologic features as soft-tissue lesions. Photomicrograph illustrates a prominent "herringbone" pattern. (Hematoxylin and eosin; x160.)

Fig. 13-5. *A,* Anteroposterior view of right proximal femur showing extensive lytic destruction secondary to fibrosarcoma. *B,* Anteroposterior view of right proximal femur after radical resection and reconstruction with a custom total hip replacement.

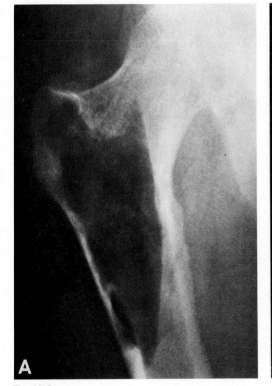
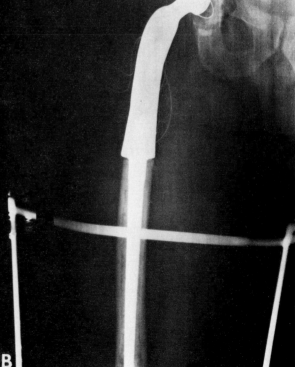

Fig. 13-5.

Treatment

Important considerations in the treatment of patients with fibrosarcoma are (1) stage of the disease at presentation, (2)

Fibrosarcoma

location, (3) extent, and (4) pathologic grade of the lesion. As outlined in Chapter 3, a careful preoperative assessment is mandatory before definitive surgical therapy is done. The general health of the patient, as well as evidence of occult systemic

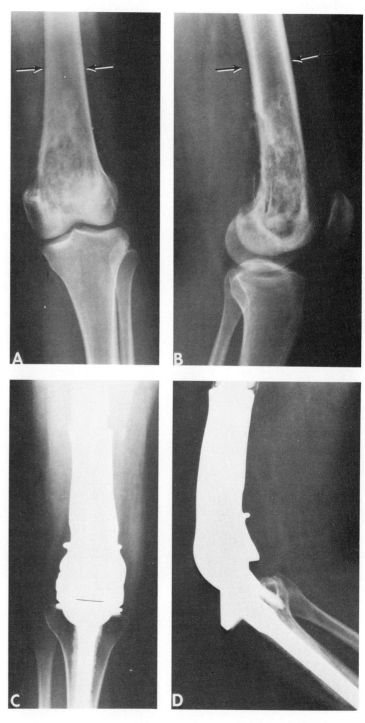

Fig. 13-6. Anteroposterior (*A*) and lateral (*B*) views of right femur showing recurrent grade 1 fibrosarcoma (*arrows*). *C* and *D*, After resection and custom prosthetic replacement.

metastasis, must be evaluated. Plain roentgenograms, bone scans, and computed tomographic scans often supplemented by angiography determine the regional extent of involvement of the tumor. When the diagnosis of a fibrosarcoma of bone, either central or peripheral, is firmly established and there is no apparent metastasis, radical surgery is indicated. Moreover, the presence of pulmonary metastasis on admission is not an absolute contraindication to radical surgery, since pulmonary resection coupled with chemotherapy may provide long-term disease-free survival. As pointed out by Enneking et al (16), the aggressiveness of the surgical approach should correlate with the surgical stage of the lesion, and amputation is most commonly recommended for patients with high-grade extraosseous lesions (stage II). The site for the amputation depends on the location and size of the tumor as determined by radiography and bone scan. The Mayo Clinic series indicates that in patients with fibrosarcoma of bone, survival rates and histologic grade are related, there being a poorer prognosis for patients with undifferentiated lesions.

If pretreatment studies indicate a low surgical stage (IA or IB), or even a stage II lesion, if it is confined to the bone, and particularly if it is small, limb-saving surgery may be effective. This would necessitate an en bloc resection, which would achieve a wide margin of bone and surrounding soft tissue (Fig. 13-5 and 13-6). The method of skeletal reconstruction will vary with the location of the tumor, as outlined in Chapter 5. A Tinkoff-Lindberg humeral interscapulo-thoracic resection may be required for proximal lesions of the upper extremity, and an internal hemipelvectomy may be needed for lesions involving the pelvis.

Radiation therapy is considered ineffective for this lesion but may have some palliative value. Adjuvant polychemotherapy programs after surgical treatment are being evaluated at our institution and at other centers in an effort to reduce the risk of fatal microscopic residual metastatic disease. Our experience indicates that fibrosarcoma of bone is more lethal than fibrosarcoma of soft tissues. Overall, 28.7% of patients survived 5 years, whereas 21.8% survived 10 years or more. As with other malignant bone tumors, this lesion demands prompt, adequate treatment and requires teamwork among all disciplines involved.

References

1. Dahlin DC: Bone Tumors: General Aspects and Data on 3,987 Cases. Second edition. Springfield, Illinois, Charles C Thomas, Publishers, 1967, pp 212–221
2. Eyre-Brook AL, Price CH: Fibrosarcoma of bone: review of fifty consecutive cases from the Bristol Bone Tumour Registry. J Bone Joint Surg [Br] 51:20–37, 1969
3. Geschickter CF: So-called fibrosarcoma of bone: bone involvement by sarcoma of the neighboring soft parts. Arch Surg 24:231–291, 1932

4. MacDonald I, Budd JW: Osteogenic sarcoma. I. A modified nomenclature and a review of 118 five year cures. Surg Gynecol Obstet 77:413–421, 1943
5. Phemister DB: Cancer of the bone and joint. JAMA 136:545–554, 1948
6. Cunningham MP, Arlen M: Medullary fibrosarcoma of bone. Cancer 21:31–37, 1968
7. Jaffe HL: Tumors and Tumerous Conditions of the Bones and Joints. Philadelphia, Lea & Febiger, 1958, pp 298–313
8. Lichtenstein L: Bone Tumors. Third edition. St Louis, CV Mosby Company, 1965, pp 229–240
9. Stout AP: Fibrosarcoma: the malignant tumor of fibroblasts. Cancer 1:30–63, 1948
10. Gilmer WS Jr, MacEwen GD: Central (medullary) fibrosarcoma of bone. J Bone Joint Surg [Am] 40:121–141, 1958
11. Dahlin DC, Ivins JC: Fibrosarcoma of bone: a study of 114 cases. Cancer 23:35–41, 1969
12. Nielsen AR, Poulsen H: Multiple diffuse fibrosarcomata of the bones. Acta Pathol Microbiol Scand 55:265–272, 1962
13. Steiner PE: Multiple diffuse fibrosarcoma of bone. Am J Pathol 20:877–893, 1944
14. Dorfman HD, Norman A, Wolff H: Fibrosarcoma complicating bone infarction in a caisson worker: a case report. J Bone Joint Surg [Am] 48:528–532, 1966
15. Morris JM, Lucas DB: Fibrosarcoma within a sinus tract of chronic draining osteomyelitis: case report and review of literature. J Bone Joint Surg [Am] 46:853–857, 1964
16. Enneking WF, Spanier SS, Goodman MA: A system for the surgical staging of musculoskeletal sarcoma. Clin Orthop 153:106–120, 1980

Chapter 14

SACROCOCCYGEAL CHORDOMA

Douglas J. Pritchard, M.D.
Krishnan K. Unni, M.B., B.S.
John W. Beabout, M.D.

Chordoma is a relatively uncommon tumor that is believed to derive from areas of primitive notochordal tissue. While this tumor may arise anywhere along the spinal column, it is most often found at the ends: at the base of the skull or at the sacrococcygeal region. About half of all chordomas occur in the sacrococcygeal region and about 35% occur at the base of the skull. Most of the remainder involve the cervical vertebrae; the dorsal and lumbar vertebrae are rarely affected. The tumor is located strictly in the midline regions of the body. Sacrococcygeal chordoma is of particular interest to the orthopedic surgeon since this tumor may cause low-back pain and since chordoma constitutes approximately 2% of all malignant tumors of bone (1,2). Chordoma is rarely encountered in patients who are less than 30 years of age. Males are more commonly affected than females.

Clinical Features

Most patients with sacrococcygeal chordoma complain of low-back or buttock pain; sometimes the pain is of many months' duration. Constipation may be a prominent complaint because the tumor is near the lower part of the rectum, and there is the possibility of nerve destruction by the tumor. Urinary frequency, urgency, or difficulty initiating urination may gradually develop. Eventually, urinary and fecal incontinence may result. In the late stages of this disease, pain may be severe and extremely difficult to manage. Chordoma found in other sites, for example, in the more cephalad portions of the spinal column, may produce symptoms from nerve compression or from the presence of a mass.

Sacrococcygeal chordomas almost always erode through the anterior surface of the sacrum and produce a presacral mass. In most cases, this mass is appreciated on rectal examination. Proctoscopic examination is useful to determine whether the lesion is extrarectal.

Unfortunately, it is not always easy to get good-quality roentgenograms of the sacrum. Hence, the tumor may be overlooked. Good-quality films may reveal an irregular zone of destruction in the central portion of the sacrum. Chordoma may produce an eccentric zone of destruction, but this is rare. Usually, there is evidence of a soft-tissue mass extending anteriorly and occasionally posteriorly. The differential diagnosis on the roentgenogram includes metastatic disease, myeloma, and giant cell tumor. Chondrosarcoma also may arise in the sacrum (Fig. 14–1).

Computed tomography (CT) is particulary helpful in determining the extent of the tumor: both the interosseous destruction and the subperiosteal presacral extension may be clearly defined. CT may be done with contrast medium so that the urinary system and the major vessels can be visualized. Technetium or gallium bone scans and chest roentgenograms also should be done to rule out the possibility of metastatic disease. It is extremely helpful to have as much information about the primary lesion as possible prior to the taking of a biopsy specimen.

Pathologic Findings

Chordoma is a soft tumor that varies in consistency from solid to almost liquid mucoid tissue. The soft-tissue extent of the presacral lesion is usually covered by periosteum. Areas of focal calcification or even ossification may be present. Even at low power, chordoma cells are characteristically arranged in lobules. Syncytial strands of cells are characteristically found lying in a mass of mucus. Physaliphorous cells with intracytoplasmic vacuoles containing mucus also are commonly found (Fig. 14-2).

Treatment

Various surgical approaches for sacral and presacral tumors have been advocated. In 1952, McCarty et al (3) described a posterior approach to these tumors. Since that report, most patients with sacral chordomas at the Mayo Clinic have been treated by this approach. Block resection with a margin of normal tissue on all aspects is ideal but difficult to achieve.

For this approach, the patient is positioned in the Kraske position, and a midline incision is made over the sacrum and coccyx. Skin flaps are fashioned, leaving normal subcutaneous tissue overlying the sacrum if the tumor extends posteriorly. Any prior wound scars or biopsy sites must be included in the resection. Care is taken at all times to avoid entering the tumor. The coccyx is usually removed separately and discarded, unless the tumor actually invades this structure. With the coccyx removed, the rectum and pelvic contents may be mobilized to protect them during later sacral resection. It may be helpful to insert a flat ribbon retractor between the sacrum and the rectum. The sacrum is osteotomized, usually at the S-3 level, unless the tumor extends more proximally. It was formerly believed that the nerve roots of S-3 need to be preserved in order to ensure adequate bowel, bladder, and sexual functions; however, currently the guiding philosophy is that the tumor should be resected completely, regardless of the number of nerve roots that need to be sacrificed. Stener and Gunterberg (4) demonstrated that if all the sacral nerves are sacrificed on one side and preserved on the other, there will be minimal functional deficit. If the upper two nerve roots on one side and the upper three on the other side can be spared, the resulting functional deficit will be manageable by most patients. If all except the upper nerve root is sacrificed bilaterally, the patient will have bowel and bladder incontinence and some loss of sexual function (4,5).

In a recent report of 50 patients who had complete wide

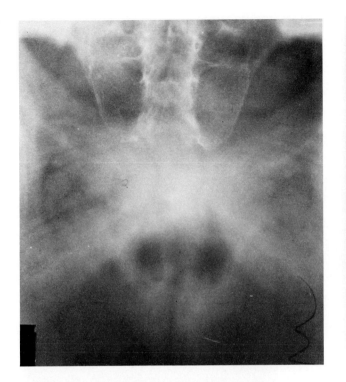

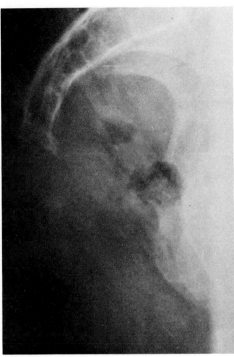

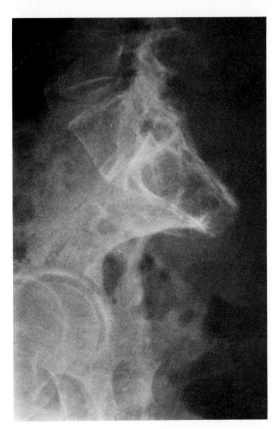

Fig. 14-1. Anteroposterior (*A*) and lateral (*B*) views of sacrum of 47-year-old man with a chordoma. Note anterior extension on lateral view. Lateral view *(C)* of after resection.

Fig. 14-1.

Sacrococcygeal Chordoma

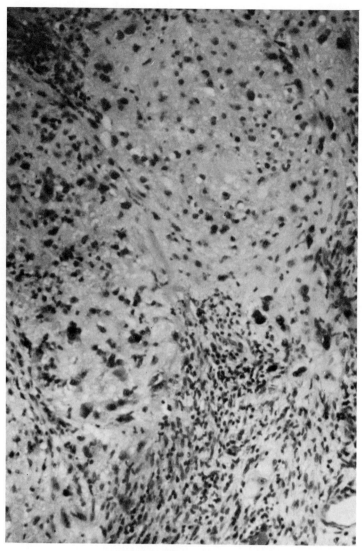

Fig. 14-2. Histologic appearance of typical chordoma. (Hematoxylin and eosin; x100.)

Fig. 14-2

excision of the tumor, 25 had clean resections without violation of the tumor at surgery (6). Of these, seven (28%) subsequently had local recurrences. However, for the 25 patients whose tumors were entered at the time of surgery, 16 (64%) had one or more local recurrences. Thus, if one is to avoid local recurrence and perhaps subsequent metastatic disease, the tumor should be completely resected at the first surgical procedure, without breaking or cutting into the tumor during the procedure. While the posterior approach allows for resection of most sacrococcygeal chordomas, some are so large that a combined anterior and posterior approach is necessary. In this case, the anterior incision is usually made by a general surgeon. The rectum is dissected away from the anterior surface of the tumor, the major vessels are isolated and protected, and the tumor and sacrum are exposed. The anterior wound can then be closed, the patient turned to the prone position, and the posterior incision made. The sacrum can then be osteotomized and the entire block of tumor-bearing tissue removed.

In advanced disease, chordoma may erode into any or all of the normal structures contained in the pelvis. The sacral and presacral nerve roots may be destroyed by the tumor. The tumor may erode into or through the bowel or bladder or may seed the peritoneum. Local or regional growth may be extensive and may cause the death of the patient. In addition to aggressive local disease, chordoma may metastasize to distant sites. It is unusual for metastasis to occur if the original lesion is cleanly resected. However, with the development of local recurrence, the possibility of distant metastasis increases greatly.

Numerous severe complications are associated with the surgery that is required for the cure of sacral chordoma. These include the possible loss of bladder, bowel, and sexual functions. However, if the surgeon does not use this radical approach, the tumor is likely to produce its own set of complications and the added risk of subsequent metastasis and death.

It is not known at this time whether radiation therapy is of value in patients with sacrococcygeal chordoma. There are not enough data in the literature or in our own experience to answer the question as to whether radiation should be used as an adjunct to surgery. We have observed that radiation treatment is sometimes a helpful palliative measure for patients with advanced disease (6–8).

References

1. Dahlin DC: Chordoma. *In* Bone Tumors: General Aspects and Data on 6,221 Cases. Third edition. Springfield, Illinois, Charles C Thomas, Publisher, 1978, pp 329–343
2. Heffelfinger MJ, Dahlin DC, MacCarty CS, et al: Chordomas and cartilaginous tumors at the skull base. Cancer 32:410–420, 1973
3. MacCarty CS, Waugh JM, Mayo CW, et al: The surgical treatment of presacral tumors: a combined problem. Proc Staff Meet Mayo Clin 27:73–84, 1952
4. Stener B, Gunterberg B: High amputation of the sacrum for extirpation of tumors: principles and technique. Spine 3:351–366, 1978
5. Gunterberg B: Effects of major resection of the sacrum: clinical studies on urogenital and anorectal function and a biomechanical study on pelvic strength. Acta Orthop Scand [Suppl] 162:1–38, 1976
6. Kaiser T, Pritchard DJ: Unpublished data.
7. Sundaresan N, Galicich JH, Chu FCH, et al: Spinal chordomas. J Neurosurg 50:312–319, 1979
8. Mindell ER: Current concepts review: chordoma. J Bone Joint Surg [Am] 63:501–505, 1981

Chapter 15

SMALL ROUND-CELL MALIGNANCIES OF BONE

Douglas J. Pritchard, M.D.
Krishnan K. Unni, M.B., B.S.
Gerald S. Gilchrist, M.D.

Lymphoma of bone, neuroblastoma metastatic to bone, and Ewing's sarcoma of bone are composed primarily of small round cells. These tumors all tend to be relatively radiosensitive; that is, they respond better to radiation treatment than do other bone sarcomas. However, each of these small round-cell tumors has its own distinct clinical, roentgenographic, and biologic behavior, and each demands consideration of different treatment modalities (1).

Lymphoma of Bone

Reticulum cell sarcoma of bone was first described by Parker and Jackson in 1939 (2). Prior to this description, the lesion was confused with Ewing's sarcoma, and most of the small round-cell tumors were grouped together. Currently, the term "lymphoma" is generally used. Most of these tumors in bone have a mixed pattern and are not made up solely of reticulum cells. The clinical features, pathologic findings, and prognosis are considerably different for patients with lymphoma than those with Ewing's sarcoma or other small round-cell tumors.

Clinical Features. As with most other bone tumors, males are affected more frequently than females. Most patients are middle-aged or elderly adults; young people are uncommonly affected. In the Mayo Clinic experience (3), the pelvis, proximal femur, rib, and distal femur are most commonly affected; however, lymphoma may arise in any bone. It may not be possible to determine whether the lesion is arising in bone, especially when the lesion is in the region of the spinal column. About 40% of all lymphomas of bone apparently are primary in bone. Careful preoperative evaluation is necessary to exclude the possibility of systemic or metastatic disease. This includes obtaining a technetium-99 bone scan, bone marrow aspiration, chest roentgenograms, and consideration of computed tomography of the abdomen and pelvis to rule out nodal or visceral disease.

Presenting Symptoms. Patients with lymphoma of bone note pain and swelling in the region of the lesion. The patient may be seen initially because of a pathologic fracture.

Laboratory Findings. In addition to a careful physical examination, one should consider the use of other diagnostic modalities, such as lymphangiography and computed tomography to help rule out nodal disease. Abdominal exploration is probably not necessary if these other modalities are utilized. In addition, bone marrow aspirates are useful to exclude the possibility of marrow involvement. Special blood smears should be studied to rule out the possibility of acute leukemia, which also may present as a primary destructive lesion of bone (4).

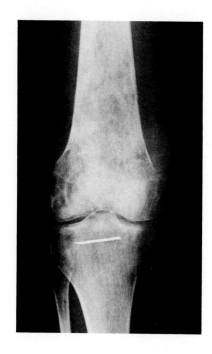

Roentgenologic Features. Lymphoma of bone usually presents with a diffuse, destructive, mottled roentgenographic appearance. There may be extensive areas of bony involvement, and the margins of the lesions tend to blend into the unaffected areas. Cortical bone is usually eroded, and the tumor may extend into the adjacent soft tissues. In some cases, cortical bone may be thickened; however, periosteal new bone formation is not as prominent as it is in Ewing's sarcoma (Fig. 15-1).

Pathologic Findings. The gross tumor tissue is gray-white and very soft. Involved bone may show extensive destruction, with areas of necrosis. Microscopically, lymphoma is usually composed of a mixture of cell types and cannot be reliably subclassified in the way that soft-tissue lymphoma can. Reticulum cells are the most frequently encountered cells. These cells are larger than those seen in Ewing's sarcoma and tend to have grooves or infolding of the nuclei. The nuclei are prominent, and the cytoplasmic borders tend to be indistinct. Lymphocytes and lymphoblasts also are usually present. While an occasional lesion may contain only one of these cell types, it is much more common to see a mixture of cell types. Reed-Sternberg cells also may be found and may dominate. These cells tend to form an alveolar pattern with cells surrounded by reticular network; reticulum stains are sometimes helpful in delineating this network. If lymphocytes are prominently present, this may lead to the erroneous diagnosis of osteomyelitis. Histiocytosis X also may be confused with lymphoma of bone, although the cells of histiocytosis X lack features suggestive of malignancy (Fig. 15-2).

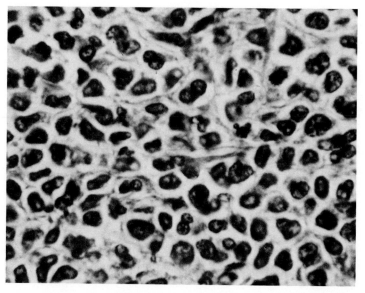

Fig. 15-1. Anteroposterior view of distal femur showing mottled destruction, typical of lymphoma.

Fig. 15-2. Typical histologic appearance of lymphoma of bone. (Hematoxylin and eosin; x650.)

Bone Tumors

Treatment. Lymphoma is a radiosensitive tumor; therefore, radiation therapy is generally employed and is usually the only treatment indicated if the clinical evaluation suggests that there is no metastatic or systemic disease present (5). There is no clear-cut or obvious advantage to the use of adjunctive chemotherapy at the time of initial treatment. However, patients with lymphoma should be followed up closely with frequent physical examinations and repeat roentgenograms or bone scans, with the expectation that chemotherapy will be utilized if systemic involvement occurs. Surgery is generally reserved for patients with pathologic fractures that cannot be reasonably managed by some other means. The surgeon's main role in this disease, then, is in the preoperative evaluation and in the establishment of the diagnosis through biopsy. Care should be taken in the performance of the biopsy to minimize the extent of dissection and to establish hemostasis. In this manner, radiation therapy may be initiated soon after the performance of the biopsy (approximately 2 to 3 weeks).

Prognosis. If the results of clinical evaluation suggest that the lesion is truly primary in bone, with no evidence of systemic involvement, the prognosis for lymphoma is generally better than for Ewing's sarcoma and most other malignant bone tumors. However, 5-year survival rates are not a valid indication of progression, since lymphoma of bone may recur and metastasize much later. No relationship exists between the site of the original involvement and the subsequent prognosis (6). This is in contrast to the situation with Ewing's sarcoma, in which the prognosis for patients with lesions of the pelvis is much worse than for those with lesions in other sites. Metastasis may occur to other bones, to regional or distant nodes, or to other soft tissues. The few patients who have essentially pure Hodgkin's or lymphocytic disease tend to have a somewhat worse prognosis (4,7).

Neuroblastoma of Bone

Neuroblastomas usually arise either in the adrenal medulla or in other sympathetic tissue. Because this tumor may metastasize to bone, it should be included in the differential diagnosis of small round-cell sarcomas. The tumor usually is seen in young children, frequently very young children. This is a very important point in the differential diagnosis; thus, if a lesion is seen in the bone of a child less than 3 years old, neuroblastoma should be suspected rather than Ewing's sarcoma or some other lesion. However, not all patients with neuroblastoma are young: adults may have this disease. Males are more frequently affected than females.

Site of Bony Metastasis. The skull is probably most often involved with metastatic skeletal disease; however, the long bones may be involved. Usually the patient has a known neuroblastoma and subsequently develops more metastatic lesions. However, a patient occasionally may present with a solitary undiagnosed bony lesion. In such a case, the roentgenographic appearance of the lesion is not specific. In fact, the lesion may mimic Ewing's sarcoma or osteomyelitis (Fig. 15-3). With widespread skeletal metastasis, there may be diffuse demineralization that resembles osteoporosis. There is a tendency for skeletal metastasis to be bilaterally symmetrical.

Pathologic Features. The histologic findings in neuroblastoma also are not always specific. While in most lesions small round cells are arranged in rosettes, this is not always true. These so-called rosettes are round aggregations of tumor cells that may be interlaced with neurofibrils; these fibrils can be difficult to demonstrate. Even if the cells of the primary site show rosettes, metastatic lesions do not always have this feature. The cells themselves are small and round, with little cytoplasm, and typically have vacuolated nuclei. Willis (8) reported on the difficulties in distinguishing Ewing's sarcoma from metastatic neuroblastoma. He described two patients who had clinical and roentgenographic features characteristic of Ewing's sarcoma; both patients ultimately were proved to have metastatic neuroblastoma (Fig. 15-4).

Laboratory Findings. The urinary excretion of catecholamines in patients with neuroblastoma is extremely helpful. Elevated values are found in patients with neuroblastoma but not in patients with Ewing's sarcoma. This feature and the fact

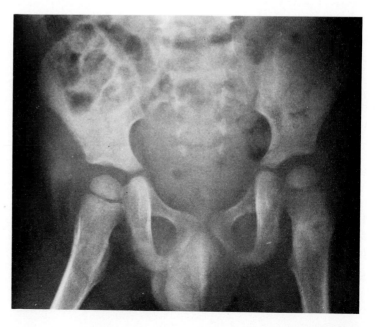

Fig. 15-3. Roentgenogram of patient with metastatic neuroblastoma. Note lesion in left proximal femur.

Bone Tumors

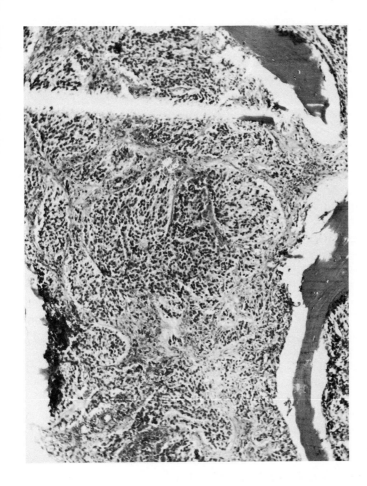

Fig. 15-4. Histologic appearance of neuroblastoma. (Hematoxylin and eosin; x100.)

that most patients with neuroblastoma are younger than patients with Ewing's sarcoma help distinguish these two diseases. From a practical standpoint, this differential diagnosis is rarely a clinical problem, as long as it is recognized that the potential for a mistake in diagnosis exists.

Orthopedic Management. Other than helping with the initial evaluation and perhaps biopsy to establish the diagnosis, orthopedists are rarely involved in the care of patients with neuroblastoma. The deformity of the spinal column which may result from radiation therapy on occasion may require orthopedic management (8–14).

Ewing's Sarcoma of Bone

This lesion was first described by Ewing (15) in 1921 and was referred to as "diffuse endothelioma of bone," but subsequently it became known as Ewing's tumor. About 5% of all malignant bone tumors are Ewing's sarcoma.

Clinical Features. As with most of the bone tumors, males are more frequently affected than females. Ewing's sarcoma is more frequent in children than in adults, although the lesion may be seen in persons of virtually any age. Very young infants, however, rarely have this tumor. This is an important differential point because young infants can have metastatic neuroblastoma.

Ewing's sarcoma occurs most frequently in bones of the pelvis and lower extremity, although any bone may be involved. Any area within a long bone may be involved, and occasionally the entire bone may be affected. The subtrochanteric region of the proximal femur is a common site.

Presenting Symptoms. Most patients experience pain that seems to become progressively worse with time, and swelling subsequently develops. Many patients have intermittent low-grade fevers. Pathologic fractures are not usually seen on presentation, although they may occur after biopsy has been done and treatment instituted. Most patients have a relatively short duration of symptoms before they seek medical attention. Patients seldom have symptoms that last more than a few months. Occasionally, a patient may have a prolonged period of symptoms before the true nature of the disease is known.

Laboratory Findings. Many patients with Ewing's sarcoma have elevated erythrocyte sedimentation rates, and some also have leukocytosis or anemia or both.

Roentgenologic Findings. The usual roentgenographic appearance is that of mottled or moth-eaten destruction containing both lytic and blastic areas. An "onionskin" appearance of the surface of the bone due to elevation of the periosteum and multiple layers of subperiosteal or active new bone formation may be seen, but this feature is not pathognomonic for Ewing's sarcoma since it may be found with other bone tumors, both benign and malignant. Any portion of a long bone may be affected; indeed, the entire bone may be involved. Usually, the extent of involvement of pathologic examination is greater than that seen on the roentgenogram. Usually, some element of bone destruction is apparent. Radiating spicules may be present on the surface of the bone, which may make the lesion indistinguishable from osteosarcoma (Fig. 15-5). The roentgenographic appearance is also similar to that seen in osteomyelitis. This similarity, combined with the finding of fever and an elevated erythrocyte sedimentation rate, may lead to the erroneous diagnosis of osteomyelitis.

Several unusual patterns are occasionally seen on the roentgenogram. The lesion may simulate a cyst, with expansion of the bone. Occasionally, the lesion involves only the surface of the bone and not the intramedullary portion of the bone. When this occurs, there may be a saucer-shaped defect in the cortical

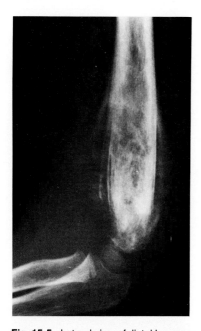

Fig. 15-5. Lateral view of distal humerus of child, showing destruction and periosteal new bone formation. Biopsy confirmed Ewing's sarcoma.

Bone Tumors

bone. This is a fairly characteristic feature of subperiosteal Ewing's sarcoma. Computed tomography may be useful in delineating the extent of the soft-tissue portion of the tumor and may provide information that is important in treatment planning. In most patients with Ewing's sarcoma, the tumor extends into the soft tissues; this may not be apparent clinically or on routine roentgenograms. In young children, the precise extent of soft-tissue involvement may be difficult to delineate even by computed tomography, since young children have proportionately less fat in their mesenchymal tissues than do older persons.

Pathologic Findings. The gross tumor tends to be white or gray and is very soft or even semiliquid. The appearance may simulate the purulence of infection. The tumor may be solid but is not encapsulated. The medullary involvement may be more extensive than is apparent on the roentgenogram. Microscopically, Ewing's sarcoma is characterized by being very cellular, the cells being remarkably similar to each other. There is usually very little stromal tissue, although bands of stroma may separate the lesion into small compartments. Individual cells are round and have round nuclei. The cell cytoplasm is usually homogeneous with indistinct cell margins. The nuclei may have a "ground-glass" appearance. Mitotic figures may be seen but are not conspicuous. Areas of extensive necrosis may be identified. Periosteal new bone formation may be present and may complicate the histologic interpretation (Fig. 15-6).

The main problem in the histologic differential diagnosis is distinguishing Ewing's sarcoma from lymphoma (16). The regularity of the cells and the nuclei, together with the lack of demonstrable reticulum, makes the usual Ewing's sarcoma relatively easy to distinguish from lymphoma. The cells of Ewing's sarcoma may contain glycogen, which may be detected by periodic acid-Schiff staining (17). However, some lesions that are Ewing's sarcoma by all other criteria do not contain glycogen, and some other tumors of bone that are clearly not Ewing's sarcoma may contain glycogen. Electron microscopy also may be helpful in the differential diagnosis; however, tumors that are equivocal by light microscopic criteria also tend to be equivocal by electron microscopy.

Nascimento et al (18) described 20 patients with large cell, "atypical" Ewing's sarcoma of bone. These patients had clinical and radiographic features characteristic of classic Ewing's sarcoma; however, histologically the cells were all or nearly all larger than those seen in Ewing's sarcoma. These cells also tended to be more polymorphic than those found in typical Ewing's tumors. These larger cells were approximately twice the size of those found in classic Ewing's tumor and were more irregular, with more prominent nuclei and more pronounced mitotic activity. These lesions must be distinguished from malignant lymphoma of bone, small cell osteosarcoma, and even metastatic adenocarcinoma. Lymphomas of bone tend to be

Small Round-Cell Malignancies of Bone

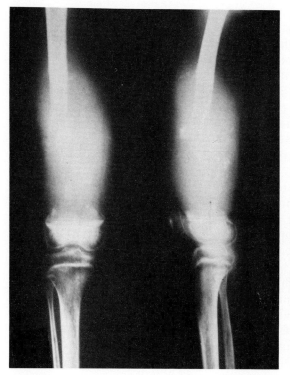 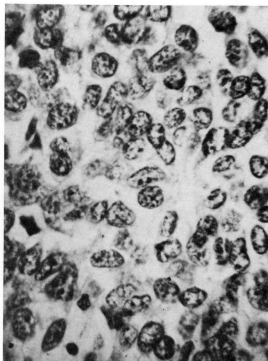

Fig. 15-6. High-power view of typical Ewing's cells. (Hematoxylin and eosin; x425.)

Fig. 15-7. Huge destructive lesion of distal femur of a child with Ewing's sarcoma, probably best treated with amputation.

much more polymorphic, with both small and large cells. In addition, the nuclei of lymphomas usually demonstrate grooving or infolding. Most lymphomas do not contain aggregates of cells in compartments, as seen in both typical and atypical Ewing's sarcoma. An additional entity that must be distinguished from Ewing's sarcoma is the recently described small cell osteosarcoma (19). The key feature of this lesion is the presence of osteoid. Metastatic neuroblastoma, rhabdomyosarcoma, and small cell carcinoma of the lungs also may be on occasion confused with Ewing's sarcoma. A complete and thorough medical evaluation is always needed to help rule out these diagnoses.

Metastasis. Ewing's sarcoma tends to metastasize to the lungs and to other bones with about equal frequency. The bones in the spinal column and skull may be involved, leading to secondary cord or brain compression. Many patients with advanced disease have neurologic symptoms and findings. While a solitary metastatic lesion may occur in the lung, showers of metastatic lesions with multiple bilateral pulmonary involvement are more common. Metastasis to regional or distant lymph nodes is unusual in Ewing's sarcoma.

Bone Tumors

Treatment. **Biopsy.** The proper planning and execution of the biopsy procedure is extremely important. The most important function of the biopsy is to provide the pathologist with an adequate, representative specimen. Open biopsy is clearly preferable to needle biopsy in the vast majority of cases. When there is soft-tissue extension of the tumor, then the biopsy specimen should be taken from that area of the tumor rather than from within the bone itself. This soft-tissue extension of the tumor tends to be easy to handle and is more representative of the tumor. The specimen should not be taken from a region where periosteal new bone formation is present, since tissue from this area may be confusing to the pathologist. The biopsy wound should be placed with the subsequent treatment in mind. Thus, if a surgical resection might be utilized for definitive treatment of the primary site, the biopsy wound should be placed so that the subsequent resection can encompass the original biopsy site. The biopsy wound should be large enough to provide adequate exposure, but the wound should be kept as small as possible. If it is necessary to violate cortical bone, a small, round hole should be made in the cortex. The tension side of the bone should be avoided whenever possible. These principles are particularly important when the lesion involves the proximal portion of the femur, where great stresses may lead to a subsequent pathologic fracture. In this situation, a small, round hole made on the anterior aspect of the greater trochanter is preferable.

When the patient presents with intermittent fever, an elevated sedimentation rate, and roentgenographic findings compatible with osteomyelitis, the surgeon may not consider Ewing's sarcoma in the differential diagnosis. He may be further misled when at biopsy the tumor has the consistency of purulence. While, in this situation, material should be obtained for culture, one also should obtain tissue for histologic examination.

Primary Lesion. Ewing's sarcoma is relatively radiosensitive. Until recently, radiation of the primary lesion was considered to be the treatment of choice for nearly all patients with Ewing's sarcoma. The dose and volume of radiation desirable for treatment are still somewhat controversial. A dose of 4,000 to 6,000 rads is generally used, with the volume covering the entire bone. It is not definitely established, however, that the entire bone needs to be treated, particularly if only one end of the long bone is involved.

Several significant problems are associated with radiation therapy. The problems include the effectiveness of radiation in controlling the primary lesion and the complications of radiation therapy. The effectiveness of radiation therapy in controlling the primary lesion is not precisely known. The tumor may recur, even many years later. If metastatic disease develops, the original primary site may not receive the same attention that it did before, and local recurrences may be overlooked. There is no reliable way to establish whether the primary lesion is completely eradicated by the original radiation treatment. Bone scans of the primary site may remain positive for more than a year. When the bone scan becomes negative and then subsequently becomes positive, this is an indication for repeat biopsy. In general, however, repeat biopsies are not routinely indicated. Biopsy might be expected to lead to a higher incidence of local complications. In addition, there could be sampling errors and small foci of cells could be missed.

Relatively little information about local recurrence is available from autopsy studies, but one such study noted what appeared to be viable tumor at the tumor site in 13 (62%) of 21 cases (20). In the recent intergroup experience on Ewing's sarcoma, 15% of the patients treated by radiation therapy had evidence of local recurrence (21). Complications of radiation therapy include severe fibrosis and soft-tissue contractures, radiation necrosis, pathologic fractures, leg-length inequality due to premature closure of epiphyses, and late radiation-induced second malignant lesions (22). Young, growing children are particularly susceptible to severe inequality of leg lengths. Some of these complications may necessitate subsequent amputation. The incidence of secondary radiation-induced malignancies is not known. With patients surviving for longer periods because of adjunctive systemic treatment, more such patients are being seen. In this situation, a new, histologically different sarcoma may arise within the field of radiation therapy 4 years or more after the original treatment.

Recently, there has been interest in surgical resection as an alternative to radiation therapy. When an expendable bone is involved with Ewing's sarcoma, surgical resection is probably preferable to radiation treatment. Thus, tumors in the ribs, fibula, and clavicle generally can be resected without significant sacrifice of function. If surgical resection of the primary lesion is utilized, careful preoperative planning is necessary to achieve optimal results. Surgery must be planned in such a way that the entire lesion can be resected with a margin of normal tissue on all aspects so that the tumor need not be entered at the time of surgery. The entire bone need not be removed as long as the lesion can be encompassed with normal histologic margins. The margins should be checked by frozen section at surgery and by permanent histologic sections. If the tumor is completely eradicated by surgery, with normal margins and without the tumor being entered, there probably is no need for radiation therapy. Radiation therapy should be used if the margins of resection are not microscopically free or if the tumor is entered at surgery.

Other approaches to the primary lesion are currently being studied. Various combination chemotherapy programs are being administered with the expectation that the primary lesion will diminish in size and thereby be more readily treated by either radiation or surgical excision. Alternatively, various combinations of chemotherapy and radiation therapy may be given before consideration of a secondary surgical excision. Considerable judgment is necessary in selecting the proper approach for a particular patient (23–27).

There are three main indications for amputation for Ewing's sarcoma: if the lesion is very large with considerable soft-tissue extension; if the patient has a pathologic fracture that cannot be managed by any other reasonable means; and if the lesion arises in the region of the distal femur or in the leg or foot of a young, growing child. In these situations, radiation therapy might produce an unacceptable limb-length inequality or poor function (Fig. 15-7).

Systemic. In recent years, adjunctive chemotherapy has been utilized in an effort to prevent metastatic disease from developing and to prolong life (28). Numerous chemotherapy programs are currently being studied. Most of these involve combinations of chemotherapeutic agents. No one treatment protocol seems to be clearly preferable. Most oncologists believe that systemic chemotherapy should be continued for at least 1 year; however, there are no convincing data available regarding the optimal length of treatment.

Prognosis and Survival. In the past, only about 15% of patients with Ewing's sarcoma survived 5 years or longer. Patients with metastatic disease almost invariably died of the disease. At the present time, 40 to 50% of patients with Ewing's sarcoma survive 5 years or longer. Patients with pelvic lesions have a particularly bad prognosis. In addition, the patient who is very young or who is a male has a worse prognosis. If a recurrence develops at the primary site, the prognosis is virtually identical to that seen with metastatic disease.

References

1. Dahlin DC: Bone Tumors: General Aspects and Data on 6,221 Cases. Third edition. Springfield, Illinois, Charles C Thomas Publisher, 1978
2. Parker F Jr, Jackson H Jr: Primary reticulum cell sarcoma of bone. Surg Gynecol Obstet 68:45–53, 1939
3. Boston HC Jr, Dahlin DC, Ivins JC, et al.: Malignant lymphoma (so-called reticulum cell sarcoma) of bone. Cancer 34:1131–1137, 1974
4. Silverstein MN, Kelly PJ: Leukemia with osteoarticular symptoms and signs. Ann Intern Med 59:637–645, 1963
5. Wang CC, Fleischli DJ: Primary reticulum cell sarcoma of bone: with emphasis on radiation therapy. Cancer 22:994–998, 1968
6. Shoji H, Miller TR: Primary reticulum cell sarcoma of bone: significance of clinical features upon the prognosis. Cancer 28:1234–1244, 1971
7. Sweet DL, Mass DP, Simon MA, et al: Histiocytic lymphoma (reticulum-cell sarcoma) of bone: current strategy for orthopaedic surgeons. J Bone Joint Surg [Am] 63:79–84, 1981
8. Willis RA: Metastatic neuroblastoma in bone presenting the Ewing syndrome, with a discussion of "Ewing's sarcoma." Am J Pathol 16:317–332, 1940
9. Fraser RD, Paterson DC, Simpson DA: Orthopaedic aspects of spinal tumours in children. J Bone Joint Surg [Br] 59:143–151, 1977
10. Mayfield JK, Riseborough EJ, Jaffe N, et al: Spinal deformity in children treated for neuroblastoma: the effect of radiation and other forms of treatment. J Bone Joint Surg [Am] 63:183–193, 1981

11. Pochedly C: Neuroblastoma. Acton, Massachusetts, Publishing Sciences Group, 1976

12. Groncy P, Finklestein JZ: Neuroblastoma. *In* Pediatric Cancer Therapy. Edited by C Pochedly. Baltimore, University Park Press, 1979, pp 125–145

13. Fernbach DJ, Williams TE, Donaldson MH: Neuroblastoma. *In* Clinical Pediatric Oncology. Second edition. Edited by WW Sutow, TJ Vietti, DJ Fernbach. St. Louis, CV Mosby Company, 1977, pp 506–537

14 Robinson R: Tumours That Secrete Catecholamines: Their Detection and Clinical Chemistry. New York, J Wiley & Sons, 1980

15. Ewing J: Diffuse endothelioma of bone. Proc NY Pathol Soc 21:17–24, 1921

16. Dahlin DC: Is it worthwhile to differentiate Ewing's sarcoma and primary lymphoma of bone? Proc Natl Cancer Conf 7:941–945, 1972

17. Schajowicz F: Ewing's sarcoma and reticulum-cell sarcoma of bone: with special reference to the histochemical demonstration of glycogen as an aid to differential diagnosis. J Bone Joint Surg [Am] 41:349–356; 362, 1959

18. Nascimento AG, Cooper KL, Unni KK, et al: A clinicopathologic study of 20 cases of large-cell (atypical) Ewing's sarcoma of bone. Am J Surg Pathol 4:29–36, 1980

19. Sim FH, Unni KK, Beabout JW, et al: Osteosarcoma with small cells simulating Ewing's tumor. J Bone Joint Surg [Am] 61:207–215, 1979

20. Telles NC, Rabson AS, Pomeroy TC: Ewing's sarcoma: an autopsy study. Cancer 41:2321–2329, 1978

21. Razek A, Perez CA, Tefft M, et al: Intergroup Ewing's sarcoma study: local control related to radiation dose, volume, and site of primary lesion in Ewing's sarcoma. Cancer 46:516–521, 1980

22. Lewis RJ, Marcove RC, Rosen G: Ewing's sarcoma—functional effects of radiation therapy. J Bone Joint Surg [Am] 59:325–331, 1977

23. Bacci G, Campanacci M, Pagani PA: Adjuvant chemotherapy in the treatment of clinically localised Ewing's sarcoma. J Bone Joint Surg [Br] 60:567–574, 1978

24. Johnson RE, Pomeroy TC: Evaluation of therapeutic results in Ewing's sarcoma. Am J Roentgenol 123:583–587, 1975

25. MacIntosh DJ, Price CHG, Jeffree GM: Ewing's tumour: a study of behaviour and treatment in forty-seven cases. J Bone Joint Surg [Br] 57:331–340, 1975

26. Pritchard DJ, Dahlin DC, Dauphine RT, et al: Ewing's sarcoma. A clinicopathological and statistical analysis of patients surviving five years or longer. J Bone Joint Surg [Am] 57:10–16, 1975

27. Chan RC, Sutow WW, Lindberg RD, et al: Management and results of localized Ewing's sarcoma. Cancer 43:1001–1006, 1979

28. Rosen G, Caparros B, Mosende C, et al: Curability of Ewing's sarcoma and considerations for future therapeutic trials. Cancer 41:888–899, 1978

CHAPTER 16

METASTATIC BONE DISEASE

Franklin H. Sim, M.D.
John H. Edmonson, M.D.
Richard A. McLeod, M.D.
Krishnan K. Unni, M.B., B.S.

The problems of metastatic bone disease are well recognized and constitute an important aspect of musculoskeletal oncology. In the skeleton, secondary neoplasms vastly outnumber primary tumors. The reported incidence of bone involvement in patients suffering from malignant neoplasms varies widely, ranging from a 12% incidence reported by Clain (1), in a series of 24,000 patients who died of cancer, to the 70% reported by Jaffe (2). Undoubtedly, the incidence of skeletal metastasis by carcinoma is greatly underestimated. The most frequently primary tumors for bone metastasis are those of the prostate, breast, kidney, thyroid, and lung. These are referred to as the osseophil or bone-seeking cancers. The less frequent (osseophobe) primary cancers are those of the skin, oral cavity, esophagus, cervix, stomach, and colon. In Clain's (1) series, the most frequent sites of bone metastasis were the vertebrae (69%), pelvis (41%), femur (25%) ribs (25%), and skull (14%); the upper extremity accounted for 20% of metastatic deposits, the humerus 9.6%, scapula 5.7%, clavicle 4.1%, radius 0.4%, and ulna and hand 0.2% each. While metastatic lesions distal to the elbow are rare, when present they are more frequently derived from the lung (2). The usual route of osseous spread of metastasizing carcinomas is by the bloodstream. The presence of Batson's (3) valveless venous system and its free communication with the venous channels of the intrathoracic abdominal viscera and chest wall explains the early occurrence of metastasis to the spinal column and pelvis from carcinoma of the prostate as well as from carcinomas of the thyroid and breast.

Evaluation

Evaluation requires careful correlation of the clinical history and examination with the laboratory tests and roentgenograms. Special studies are often indicated. Usually, metastatic bone disease is not difficult to diagnose. In a patient with a history of previous carcinoma and localized findings of pain and disability, a metastatic deposit must be suspected. The pain may be present for several months before roentgenographic changes are visible. Therefore, a patient more than 40 years of age who complains of severe bone pain, particularly in the spinal column, and who has a history of a previous malignancy must be considered to have metastatic spread until proved otherwise, despite negative findings on the roentgenograms.

As soon as the bone lesion is identified, a brief initial search for other signs of cancer is useful, including a careful history and physical examination plus a routine laboratory profile and roentgenography. The correlation of these findings usually will reveal the primary lesion. The hematologic evaluation, including serum protein determinations and marrow aspiration, may help to exclude leukemia, lymphoma, and myeloma, which may be confused with metastatic disease. The laboratory evaluation, however, is usually nonspecific. Often there is a normocytic anemia with considerable elevation of the sedimentation rate; the serum calcium level is elevated in about 10% of patients with metastasis from carcinoma of the breast, lung, and kidney. The serum acid phosphatase level is usually elevated in metastatic prostate carcinoma. An elevated serum alkaline phosphatase level may indicate that large areas of bone destruction are undergoing osseous repair. Roentgenographically, although prostate carcinomas are usually blastic, most metastatic cancers are seen as irregularly shaped osteolytic lesions with a variable osteoblastic response. Approximately 50% of the medullary region needs to be destroyed before a lesion is visible on the roentgenogram. While it is usually impossible to determine the primary site of the given carcinoma from the roentgenographic appearance of the skeletal metastasis, renal cell carcinoma frequently causes a pronounced ballooning or expansion of the bone. This expansion also can be seen in thyroid cancer, lung cancer, and primary bone tumors. Moreover, a single focus of metastatic carcinoma may be difficult to distinguish from a primary malignant tumor of bone, particularly if the source of the carcinoma is occult (Fig. 16-1).

A challenging diagnostic situation emerges, which is not uncommon in hypernephroma, rare in prostatic cancer, and occasional in thyroid cancer. However, one should have a high index of suspicion if the patient is more than 40 years of age. Conventional roentgenograms and bone scans utilizing isotopes are the two major modalities for evaluating cases of known or suspected skeletal metastasis. These two studies may be used in combination with or without tomography if the individual case warrants. In more than 90% of the cases, multiple osseous lesions will be demonstrated on the roentgenographic skeletal survey and bone scan. Computed tomography has no large role in the evaluation of patients with metastatic lesions, because the plain roentgenogram and isotope scan usually provide sufficient information. However, computed tomography is particularly helpful in areas that may be difficult to see on the roentgenogram, such as the scapula, sternum, ribs, and sacrum (Fig. 16-2).

Biopsy

Biopsy should be done early in the course of the workup to guide the clinical investigation. Even if a known primary carcinoma exists, unless the relationship with the osseous lesion is obvious, a biopsy specimen should be taken before treatment is begun. This approach has considerable therapeutic significance when one considers the response of breast, prostate, thyroid, and other cancers to hormonal manipulation. The planning and technique of the biopsy are just as important in metastatic cancer as in primary lesions of bone, particularly since a definitive surgical procedure is often contemplated or radiation therapy is planned. Moreover, it is important to minimize the

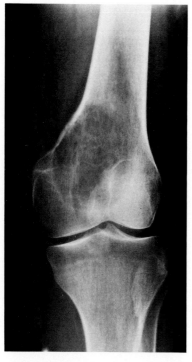

Fig. 16-1. Anteroposterior view of distal femur showing lytic lesion. Lesion has radiographic appearance of giant cell tumor but proved to be a metastatic hypernephroma from an occult primary cancer.

Bone Tumors

possibility of a pathologic fracture occurring because of the taking of a biopsy specimen, particularly in weight-bearing bone. If a metastatic hypernephroma is suspected, a biopsy specimen should not be taken unless preparation for massive loss of blood is made. The needle biopsy technique (4,5) is particularly useful in confirming known metastatic lesions and, because of the de-

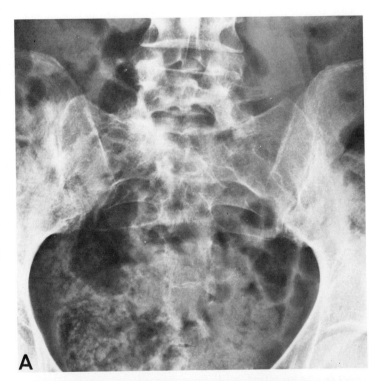

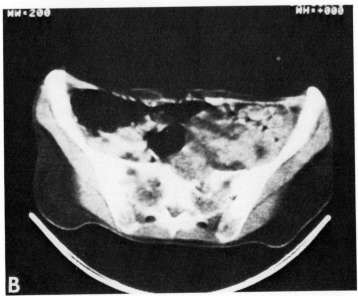

Fig. 16-2. *A*, Anteroposterior view of sacrum of patient with metastatic cancer. Lesion is not apparent. However, the CT scan of the sacrum (*B*) shows destructive lesion secondary to metastatic cancer. (*A* from Sim FH: Metastatic bone disease and myeloma. *In* Surgery of the Musculoskeletal System. Edited by CM Evarts. New York, Churchill Livingstone [in press]. By permission of Longman/Churchill Livingstone.)

Metastatic Bone Disease

creased morbidity, is most useful in lesions involving the spinal column (Fig. 16-3).

Pathologic Features

Almost all metastatic lesions to bone are of epithelial origin (Fig. 16-4). Carcinomas of the kidney, lung, breast, and prostate in particular have a propensity to metastasize to bone. Grossly, metastatic carcinomas vary from firm (secondary to a desmoplastic reaction) to soft and mushy. Histologically, most metastatic carcinomas are easily recognized as such. However, some carcinomas have a very pronounced spindling component and may be mistaken for fibrosarcomas. Sarcomatoid hypernephroma is particularly notorious in this respect. Most often some areas of the tumor will show areas of clear cells, indicating the epithelial nature of the tumor. Whenever a spindling neoplasm of bone is encountered in an older patient, the possibility of metastatic renal cell carcinoma should be considered and ruled out with appropriate diagnostic studies. Other metastatic high-grade undifferentiated carcinomas may resemble primary hemangioendotheliosarcoma of bone. Periodic acid-Schiff or mucin stains occasionally may be helpful in this differential diagnostic problem. Electron microscopy also may rarely be helpful in differentiating high-grade metastatic sarcomatoid carcinomas from primary sarcoma of bone.

Treatment Considerations

One must avoid the emotional response of hopelessness which clouds the diagnosis of metastatic bone cancer, if the quality of life remaining is to be made functional. Recognition of the full therapeutic potential of each situation is essential. This usually requires a team effort, with close cooperation among multidisciplinary groups, in order to provide logical and intelligent total management of the patient.

Medical and Radiation Management. Attention to the general status of the patient, his nutritional status, and correction of metabolic problems is important. Depending on the location and extent of bone disease, localized symptoms may be controlled by analgesics and other drugs. Various physical therapy modalities, splinting, and protection of the area may be helpful. The slowly developing fracture of metastatic origin is usually not associated with significant displacement. This slow process permits fractures of some long bones that are not involved with weight-bearing to be managed by slings, bandages, and splints. Metastatic fractures of the clavicle can be effectively treated with a figure-of-eight bandage.

The main treatment modality of the osseous metastatic lesion is radiation, the principal indication being to relieve pain and maintain or regain some useful functional activity. Radiation therapy of metastatic malignant bone disease is usually effective in controlling pain, as well as in stopping the local destructive process. Effective palliation is observed in 80% of the cases. The duration of response is variable, but generally with breast and prostate cancers, it can be for 9 to 12 months. In addition,

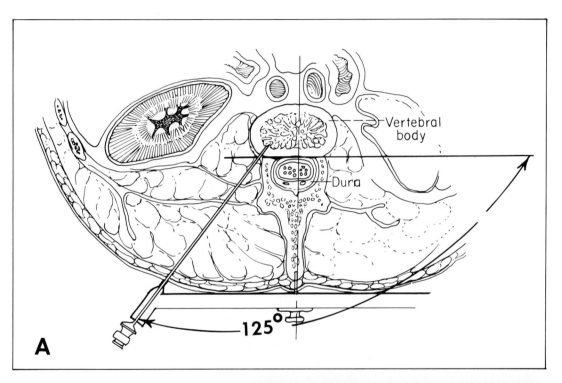

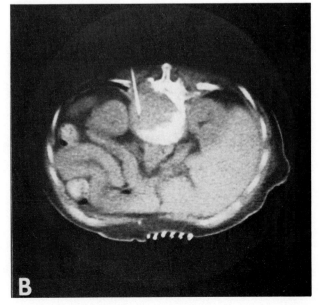

Fig. 16-3. *A,* Diagrammatic illustration of needle biopsy procedure for lumbar spinal column. The guide needle is inserted at 6.5 cm from the spinous process and angled at 125° under the image-intensifier control. When the needle is in proper position against the vertebral body, the larger biopsy needle is advanced over the exploring needle until it touches the vertebrae and is then advanced into the vertebral body. Accurate placement of the needle is facilitated by the use of CT scanning techniques (*B*). (From Sim FH: Metastatic bone disease and myeloma. *In* Surgery of the Musculoskeletal System. Edited by CM Evarts. New York, Churchill Livingstone [in press]. By permission of Longman/Churchill Livingstone.)

systemic treatment may control the neoplastic growth process and produce bone healing in some cases. This includes the use of cytotoxic drugs (6), hormonal agents, and endocrine manipulation by surgery (7), as well as radionuclide treatment (8).

Surgical Management. With improvements in medical management, patients with metastatic bone disease are surviving longer. Although the attitude of the treating physician in the past has often been conservative because of a limited life span and the generally debilitated state of the patient, an aggressive attitude must be maintained toward the treatment of these patients if symptoms are to be relieved and the quality of life is to be improved.

Intractable Pain. Persistent pain despite local and systemic therapeutic measures is a tragic problem. In recent years, improvement in the technique of percutaneous cordotomy (9) has offered hope for relief of intractable pain in these patients. As a result, amputation is rarely indicated, particularly with improvements in local management of the metastatic deposit (8). Although such radical surgery for palliative purposes seems in-

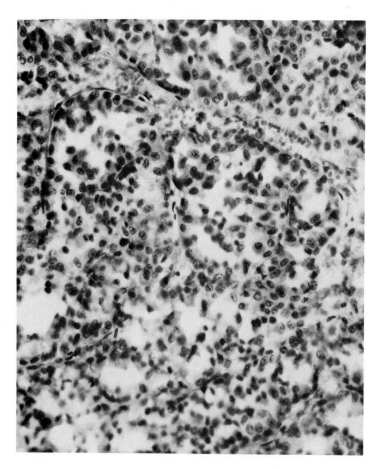

Fig. 16-4. Hypernephroma. Metastatic adenocarcinomas and renal cell carcinomas may be well differentiated. Other poorly differentiated tumors may mimic the appearance of primary bone tumors. (Hematoxylin and eosin: x400.)

Bone Tumors

congruent, the remarkable improvement of the patient with a painful fungating lesion in the shoulder girdle—for instance, with secondary infection that does not respond to medical or surgical management—occasionally may justify this procedure. At other times, particularly with lesions involving the soft tissue or an expendable bone such as the scapula, local surgical debulking may reduce the systemic effects of the tumor burden in addition to achieving pain relief. Others have advocated cryosurgery (10,11) for the surgical control of the metastatic lesion, particularly hypernephroma.

Vertebral Involvement. For pathologic fractures due to metastatic disease in the vertebrae, surgical treatment may be indicated. However, in patients with spinal metastasis and compression fracture without neurologic involvement, the intractable pain usually responds well to radiation therapy and bracing techniques.

With advanced destruction of a vertebral body and associated instability in the cervical region, immobilization in a halo cast, followed by radiation therapy, usually provides comfort and stability.

For spinal metastasis with associated neurologic involvement, decompressive laminectomy may be indicated, but usually this is helpful only before paraplegia becomes established. With laminectomy in that circumstance, stabilization of the spinal column is rarely required, except in the cervical region (Fig. 16-5). There, resection of the vertebral body (relieving the compression) and anterior fusion may be beneficial.

Pathologic Fractures. While the management of pathologic fractures should be individualized, maintenance of an aggressive program of fracture management in these circumstances does provide significant benefit (12). The principle of internal fixation has long been accepted (13–19).

In the past, many patients have been denied the benefits of internal fixation because the bone destruction seemed so extensive that it was felt that internal fixation would not succeed. However, during the past decade, it has been shown that, by combining intramedullary methyl methacrylate with an internal-fixation device, secure fixation can be achieved in most patients with extensive lesions. Moreover, the previous discouraging rate of union has been significantly improved (12,20). Most of these lesions require radiation therapy; and radiation doses as low as 2,000 rads, while they prevent tumor progression of the site of a pathologic fracture, also will prevent bone union unless rigid internal fixation has been accomplished previously (20). Consequently, healing is potentiated when rigid internal fixation is achieved by combining methyl methacrylate and internal fixation.

Prophylactic Fixation. Prophylactic internal fixation can be done when a metastatic lesion in the long bones becomes painful because of microfractures in the weakened cortex. Radiotherapy alone often will not relieve the pain; in this situation, prophylactic internal fixation should be considered before fracture

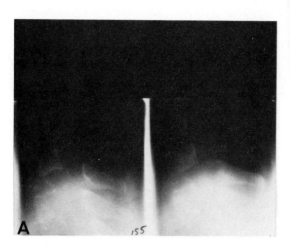
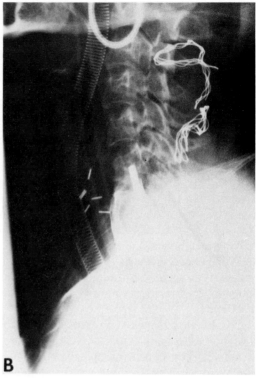

Fig. 16-5. *A*, Lateral tomograms of cervical spinal column showing extensive destruction of C-7 secondary to metastatic breast cancer. *B*, Intraoperative lateral roentgenogram of cervical spinal column showing stabilization achieved by methyl methacrylate and a Steinmann pin after excision of the vertebral body.

occurs (12,19). This technique is advocated when there are well-defined lytic lesions—those more than 3 cm in diameter in which 50% or more of the cortex is destroyed. Moreover, pain persisting in the lytic focus after treatment, regardless of the radiographic appearance, may be an indication. Prophylactic fixation before pathologic fracture occurs avoids the acute distress of the pathologic fracture, prevents displacement of the fracture fragments, and eliminates the necessity of an emergency operation. Moreover, the likelihood of such a lesion undergoing bony healing is greater than if a pathologic fracture had been allowed to occur.

Surgical Techniques. The surgical technique will vary, depending on the location of the fracture, the extent of bone destruction, and the general condition of the patient. In our previous review of the Mayo Clinic experience (12,21), 97 patients who had 102 pathologic fractures were treated by local tumor resection and open reduction and internal fixation supplemented with intramedullary methyl methacrylate (22). That review was part of a large multicenter study involving 346 patients with one or more malignant neoplastic fractures or impending fractures treated with this technique (20). In that series, the femur was involved in 274 instances, the humerus in 68, the acetabulum in 38, the tibia in 36, and the proximal ulna in 2. A major criterion for qualification for this surgical management is a life expectancy justifying the procedure, preferably 3 months. Poor quality of bone proximal and distal to the fracture is not a contraindication.

Hip and Proximal Femur Fractures. In fractures involving the head and neck of the femur, resection with prosthetic replacement is the procedure of choice. This technique is effective in achieving pain relief and early mobilization and restoration of function. The surgical technique utilizes a standard lateral approach to the hip, detaching the anterior third of the gluteus medius. While previously, extensive destruction of the calcar or lateral cortex often precluded arthroplasty, the mechanical continuity may be restored with a strong column of methyl methacrylate, ensuring complete filling of the space between the stem of the prosthesis and the surrounding cortex of bone. We used a Thompson prosthesis more commonly in the past but now find that the Bateman bipolar prosthesis gives better functional results (Fig. 16-6). Total hip arthroplasty is

Fig. 16-6. *A,* Anteroposterior view of right proximal femur showing extensive destructive lesion with pathologic fracture secondary to metastatic breast cancer. *B,* After insertion of Bateman bipolar prosthesis. (From Sim FH: Pathologic fractures. Orthop Surg Weekly Update J [in press]. By permission.)

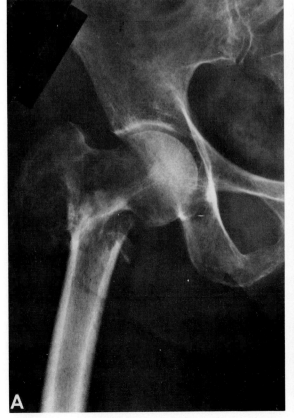 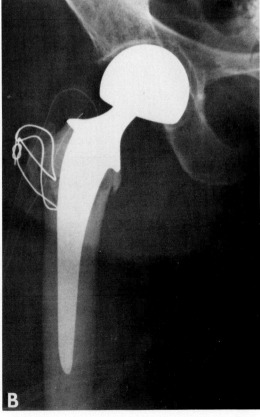

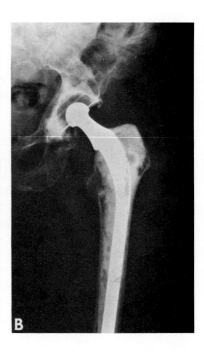

Fig. 16-7. *A,* Anteroposterior view of proximal femur and hemipelvis showing extensive destruction secondary to metastatic breast cancer. There is a pathologic fracture of the femoral neck. *B,* After long-stem Charnley total hip arthroplasty. (From Sim FH, Hartz CR, Chao EYS: Total hip arthroplasty for tumors of the hip. Hip 4:251, 1976. By permission of the C. V. Mosby Company.)

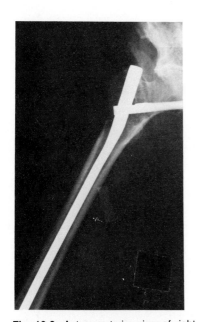

Fig. 16-8. Anteroposterior view of right proximal femur showing extensive destructive lesion in trochanteric and subtrochanteric areas secondary to metastatic breast cancer. Zickel nail has been used for fixation.

reserved for patients who are very active and are well controlled in medical management and who might benefit from the better or early functional restoration afforded by total joint replacement. Moreover, associated acetabular disease may be an indication for total hip arthroplasty. A long, straight-stem femoral prosthesis is recommended when the adjacent femoral shaft is metastatically involved (Fig. 16-7).

Intratrochanteric and subtrochanteric fractures may be managed by various techniques. A nail-plate apparatus is favored when the integrity of the proximal fragment allows secure fixation. This apparatus also offers prophylaxis against the possibility of another fracture subsequently occurring in the femoral neck. However, advocates of fixation of a subtrochanteric fracture by an intramedullary rod believe that it offers better support to the femoral shaft in the event of subsequent extension of tumor distally. In lesions of this area, a Zickel (23) nail, utilizing the standard technique, is preferred (Fig. 16-8). Moreover, prophylactic internal fixation of lesions in this region may be achieved by the use of Ender's rods (24), with minimal morbidity in very debilitated patients. Resection of the lesion and prosthetic replacement may be indicated when extensive tumor involvement proximal to the fracture creates a high risk of late failure of fixation. Our group has been encouraged by the results in 14 patients with extensive metastatic destruction of the proximal femur who had resection and segmental replacement.

Mid and Distal Femur Fractures. In one combined series (25), there were 43 fractures and 18 impending fractures of the femoral diaphysis and distal metaphysis. Internal fixation with

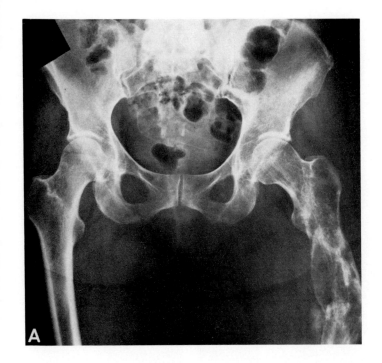

A

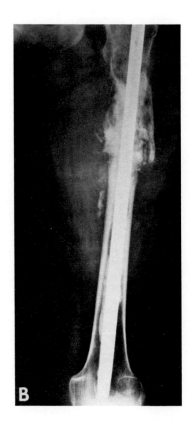

B

Fig. 16-9. *A*, Anteroposterior view of left femur showing pathologic fracture with extensive destruction secondary to metastatic breast cancer. *B*, Anteroposterior view of femur showing secure fixation with Küntscher rod combined with methyl methacrylate. (From Sim FH: Metastatic bone disease and myeloma. *In* Surgery of the Musculoskeletal System. Edited by CM Evarts. New York, Churchill Livingstone [in press]. By permission of Longman/Churchill Livingstone.)

an intramedullary rod was the procedure of choice and was performed in 44 cases (Fig. 16-9). In this technique, a standard lateral approach to the femoral shaft is utilized, and the rod is inserted in a retrograde fashion after the medullary canal has been filled with methyl methacrylate. We prefer to use a Küntscher rod. Closed rodding may be done, and this is the usual technique when this procedure is performed prophylactically. In addition, the multicenter group has surgically repaired 10 fractures of the distal femoral metaphysis. Six patients obtained secure fixation from the installation of an angle condylar blade plate and two from the use of an intramedullary rod; two with extensive destruction underwent resection and utilization of a custom hinge knee prosthesis to replace the distal femur (26).

Tibial Fractures. In patients with metastatic involvement of the tibia, prevention of a pathologic fracture may be achieved by utilization of a short leg brace. However, with extensive destruction and actual or imminent pathologic fracture, internal fixation using an intramedullary rod is recommended. A Lottes nail is preferred for this purpose (Fig. 16-10). In one series (20), 28 patients with tibial fractures underwent internal fixation and 8 with proximal lesions had prosthetic knee replacement.

Humeral Fractures. Many humeral fractures may be treated by closed means. Indications for open reduction and fixation include failure of the fracture to heal after conservative management, pain, and in many instances, the necessity of using the arms for crutch walking or supported ambulation when metastatic disease involves the spinal column or lower extremities.

Metastatic Bone Disease

Fig. 16-10. *A*, Anteroposterior view of tibia after internal fixation of right tibia with extensive metastatic cancer. Fracture line is visible. *B*, After lesions were packed with methyl methacrylate for added fixation.

Fig. 16-11. *A*, Anteroposterior humerus showing midshaft destructive lesion secondary to metastatic cancer. *B*, Surgical photograph after exteriorization of the tumor cavity and removal of tumor. *C*, Surgical photograph showing testing fit of the Rush rod across the tumor site. Methyl methacrylate is inserted into the tumor cavity and proximal distal marrow cavity, and the Rush rod is reinserted while the methacrylate is soft. *D*, Anteroposterior view of left humerus after internal fixation with Rush rod and methyl methacrylate. (*A* and *D* from Sim FH: Pathologic fractures. Orthop Surg Weekly Update J [in press]. By permission.)

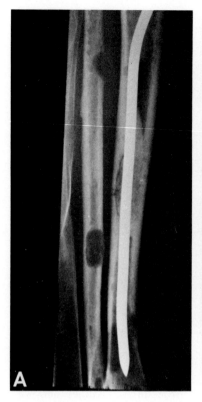
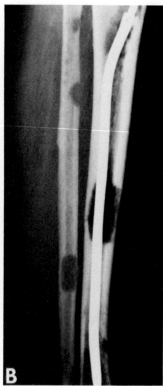

In the multicenter study (20), 68 patients were treated surgically. Three patients with extensive lytic destruction of the humeral head and neck underwent resection and proximal humeral replacement. Five patients had resection of a humeral lesion with shortening of the bone and fixation with a compression plate and methyl methacrylate. This approach may be considered when there is a small solitary metastatic deposit from a hypernephroma and the aim is potential cure rather than palliation. Our preferred technique is to utilize one or two Rush rods for internal fixation (27).

Pathologic Fractures of Long Bone. For pathologic fractures due to metastatic disease, installation of an intramedullary rod is usually the procedure of choice (Fig. 16-11). The technique varies, depending on the bone involved. In the humerus, the rod is inserted routinely through a small proximal incision that penetrates the articular margin of the humerus just posterior to the greater tubercle. After exposure of the fracture site through a lateral incision, the tumor cavity is excavated, with care to preserve remaining stable bone. The ideal length and diameter of the rod is then confirmed by roentgenographic examination, and the rod is pulled back across the fracture site into the proximal fragment. Methyl methacrylate is packed into the proximal and distal fragments and into the tumor defect; and while the methacrylate is still soft, the intramedullary rod is driven across

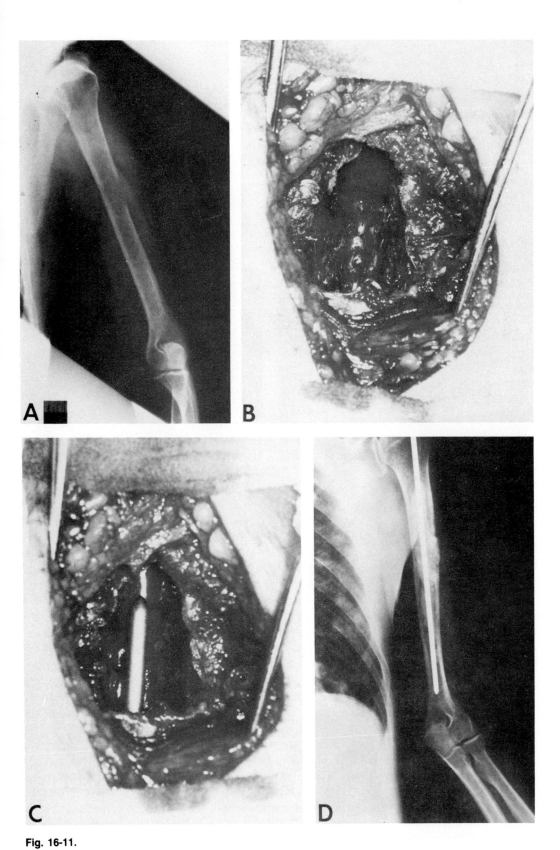

Fig. 16-11.

Metastatic Bone Disease

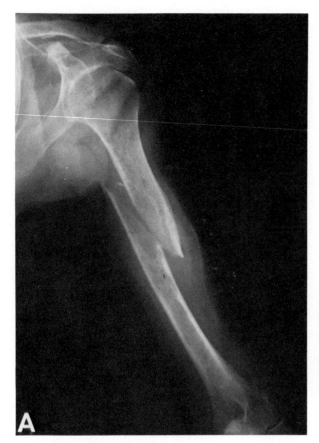
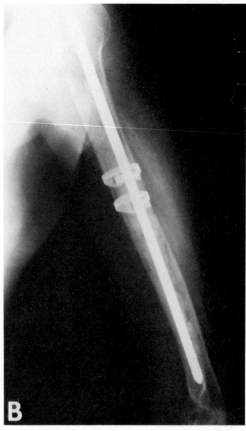

Fig. 16-12. Anteroposterior view of left humerus before (*A*) and after (*B*) internal fixation of pathologic fracture with a Rush rod and intermedullary methyl methacrylate. Two Parham bands provide additional fixation. (*A* from Sim FH, Pritchard DJ: Metastatic disease in the upper extremity. Clin Orthop 169:90, 1982. By permission of J. B. Lippincott Company.)

the fracture site into the distal fragment. Methacrylate is then used to restore the lost cortex. Care must be taken to ensure complete seating of the rod in order to avoid impingement on the acromion.

Because of the diversity of the fractures encountered, the surgical procedure may differ from the standard approach described. Besides the acrylic, two rods may be utilized to provide better rotational stability; and in spiral fractures, two Parham bands may be helpful (Fig. 16-12). For distal lesions, a posterior approach is used to obtain exposure and two Rush rods are inserted, one from each epicondyle, ensuring that the tumor cavity is filled with methyl methacrylate (Fig. 16-13).

When a plate is attached to the shaft of a long bone, the usual technique is to pack the methacrylate in the proximal and distal canals and the tumor cavity after the plate has been applied (Fig. 16-14). However, if the fixation device obstructs the insertion of the methacrylate, the device can be inserted before completion of the plating, and the remaining screws can be drilled through the hardened methacrylate after polymerization.

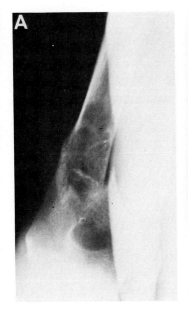
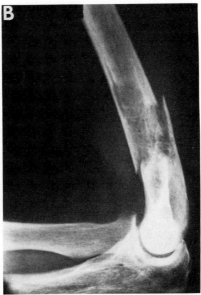
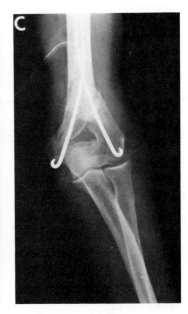

Postoperative Management

The assessment of the results of operative intervention in these patients who soon die of their disease is often difficult and at times seems to be philosophical. However, with the achievement of a stable extremity and the subsequent reduction in pain and improvement in function, the mental outlook of the patient is much improved.

In the multicenter series (20), most of the 346 patients benefited from the fixation or prosthetic replacement, obtaining both pain relief and improved mobility. Relief of pain was judged excellent or good in 85%, fair in 12%, and poor in 3%. Moreover, of the 249 patients who were ambulatory before their fractures, 233 (94%) regained the ability to walk after the operation. This compares favorably with the results reported by Parrish and Murray (19), who utilized conventional internal-fixation methods: only 52% regained ability to walk postoperatively, and after fracture fixation rather than prosthetic replacement, only 9% regained the ability to bear weight fully.

In the series from the multicenter study (20), for the 210 patients who were eligible for postoperative follow-up of 2 years or longer, the mean survival time was 14.4 months and the median 9.8 months. Among those with primary carcinoma of the breast, the mean survival was 19.8 months and the median 12.2 months. Indeed, 66% of the patients survived more than 1 year, and 38% survived more than 18 months postoperatively. Fourteen of the 210 patients were alive at 2 years, and 10 were alive at 3 years. These survival statistics are superior to those

Fig. 16-13. Anteroposterior (A) and lateral (B) views showing destructive lesion of distal humerus secondary to metastatic thyroid cancer. Anteroposterior (C) view of distal humerus showing internal fixation with two Rush rods inserted retrograde from each epicondyle, combined with intramedullary methyl methacrylate. (From Sim FH: Metastatic bone disease and myeloma. *In* Surgery of the Musculoskeletal System. Edited by CM Evarts. New York, Churchill Livingstone [in press]. By permission of Longman/Churchill Livingstone.)

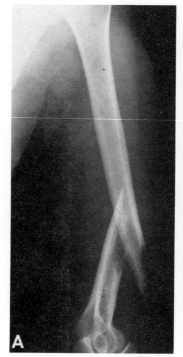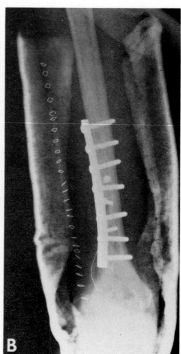

Fig. 16-14. *A*, Lateral view showing fracture of distal humerus secondary to metastatic cancer. *B*, After internal fixation with a plate, internal fragmentary screws, and methyl methacrylate.

from series using conventional fixation techniques (19) and reflect the advantage of immediate fracture stabilization and resumption of early ambulation—not to mention relief from fracture pain.

The postoperative management is individualized, depending on the location of the lesion. In lesions of the lower extremity, full weight-bearing as tolerated is encouraged within a few days of operation in order to get early and maximal independence from external support. In lesions involving the humerus, a Velpeau dressing is utilized for the first 3 days, after which mobilization and strengthening exercises are initiated. Five to 7 days after surgery, the patient is encouraged to begin using the arm in everyday activities. Most patients receive radiation therapy (approximately 3,000 rads) to the site, beginning 10 days after surgery, and later are given additional treatment, depending on the tumor type.

Conclusion

In metastatic disease, each patient should be considered individually, and the decision of the best method of treatment should be made after thorough evaluation. Although treatment of metastatic bone disease is palliative, it is important to avoid a nihilistic attitude. Good judgment must be used in deciding treatment objectives, methods, and approaches, and this usually requires a team effort. While maintenance of an aggressive approach to pathologic fractures can extend a functional life for more than a year, the physician must remember the palliative nature and goals of treatment. The goals of internal fixation are limited. In general, they are to relieve pain, improve function, and facilitate medical and nursing care.

References

1. Clain A: Secondary malignant disease of bone. Br J Cancer 19:15–29, 1965
2. Jaffe HL: Tumors and Tumorous Conditions of the Bones and Joints. Philadelphia, Lea & Febiger, 1958
3. Batson OV: The role of the vertebral veins in metastatic processes. Ann Intern Med 16:38–45, 1942
4. Craig FS: Metastatic and primary lesions of bone. Clin Orthop 73:33–38, 1970
5. Schajowicz F, Derqui JC: Puncture biopsy in lesions of the locomotor system: review of results in 4050 cases, including 941 vertebral punctures. Cancer 21:531–548, 1968
6. Chlebowski RT, Block JB: Chemotherapy of bone metastasis (II). In Bone Metastasis. Vol 4. Edited by L Weiss, HA Gilbert. Boston, GK Hall & Company, 1981, pp 312–324
7. Van Scoy-Mosher MB: Hormonal therapy of metastatic bone disease. In Bone Metastasis. Vol 4. Edited by L Weiss, HA Gilbert. Boston, GK Hall & Company, 1981, pp 325–347
8. Tong ECK: Parathormone and ^{32}P therapy in prostatic cancer with bone metastases. Radiology 98:343–351, 1971
9. Onofrio BM: Recent results with percutaneous cordotomy. Mayo Clin Proc 45:689–694, 1970
10. Marcove RC, Miller TR: The treatment of primary and metastatic localized bone tumors by cryosurgery. S Clin North Am 49:421–430, 1969
11. Marcove RC, Sadrieh J, Huvos AG, et al: Cryosurgery in the treatment of solitary or multiple bone metastases from renal cell carcinoma. J Urol 108:540–547, 1972
12. Sim FH, Daugherty TW, Ivins JC: The adjunctive use of methylmethacrylate in fixation of pathological fractures. J Bone Joint Surg [Am] 56:40–48, 1974
13. Altman H: Intramedullary nailing for pathological impending and actual fractures of long bones. Bull Hosp Joint Dis 13:239–251, 1952
14. Coley BL, Sharp GS: Pathological fractures in primary bone tumors of the extremities. Am J Surg 9:251–263, 1930
15. Devas MB, Dickson JW, Jelliffe AM: Pathological fractures: treatment by internal fixation and irradiation. Lancet 2:484–487, 1956
16. Fidler M: Prophylactic internal fixation of secondary neoplastic deposits in long bones. Br Med J 1:341–343, 1973
17. Koskinen EVS, Nieminen RA: Surgical treatment of metastatic pathological fracture of major long bones. Acta Orthop Scand 44:539–549, 1973
18. MacAusland WR Jr, Wyman ET Jr: Mangement of metastatic pathological fractures. Clin Orthop 73:39–51, 1970
19. Parrish FF, Murray JA: Surgical treatment for secondary neoplastic fractures: a retrospective study of ninety-six patients. J Bone Joint Surg [Am] 52:665–686, 1970
20. Harrington KD, Sim FH, Enis JE, et al: Methylmethacrylate as an adjunct in internal fixation of pathological fractures: experience with three hundred and seventy-five cases. J Bone Joint Surg [Am] 58:1047–1055, 1976
21. Sim FH, Ivins JC, Pritchard DJ: Management of pathological fractures at the Mayo Clinic. Ital J Orthop Traumatol [Suppl] 1:185–195, 1975

22. Dahlin DC: Bone Tumors: General Aspects and Data on 6,221 Cases. Third edition. Springfield, Illinois, Charles C Thomas, Publisher, 1978

23. Zickel RE: An intramedullary fixation device for the proximal part of the femur: nine years' experience. J Bone Joint Surg [Am] 58:866–872, 1976

24. Pankovich AM, Tarabishy IE: Ender nailing of intertrochanteric and subtrochanteric fractures of the femur: complications, failures, and errors. J Bone Joint Surg [Am] 62:635–645, 1980

25. Sim FH, Chao EYS: Prosthetic replacement of the knee and a large segment of the femur or tibia. J Bone Joint Surg [Am] 61:887–892, 1979

26. Lewallen RP, Pritchard DJ, Sim FH: Treatment of pathologic fractures or impending fractures of the humerus with Rush rods and methylmethacrylate: experience with 55 cases in 54 patients, 1968–1977. Clin Orthop 166:193–198, 1982

CHAPTER 17

REHABILITATION

Henry H. Stonnington, M.B., B.S., M.SC.

The diagnosis of a bone tumor or widespread metastasis is a catastrophic event in the lives of the patient and family. The use of rehabilitative techniques not only will teach them to change their life-styles but also will improve the quality of life by fulfilling many needs. The techniques that are available to any institution or medical practice are cost-effective and are as important as surgery, radiation, or chemotherapy in the general management of these patients. The proper use of prosthetics is part of the management. It is assumed that the reader has knowledge of this topic or has access to texts on the subject (1), and this area will not be discussed to any extent. This chapter is primarily devoted to the methods needed to improve the quality of life—for example, the prevention of a prosthesis becoming a handicap.

An impairment, a disability, and a handicap are different. An impairment is an abnormality or a disturbance of an organ, for example, an amputated limb. A disability is the consequence of an impairment in that the impairment restricts the activity and function of the patient. For example, although the amputee may be able to ambulate well, the fact that the patient has a limb missing makes him feel abnormal and different. This feeling may prevent the patient from engaging in the ordinary activities of life. A handicap concerns the disadvantages experienced by the patient as a result of the impairment and disability, reflecting the lack of adaptation to the patient's surroundings (2). Thus, the handicapped amputee feels that he cannot fulfill the role that he had before the tumor was discovered. Many prior psychologic and social factors are important in the determination of a handicap (Fig. 17-1).

As soon as the patient reaches the stage of being handicapped, a vicious cycle begins in that the patient feels deprived not only of basic physical needs but also of psychologic needs (3) (Fig. 17-2). The resulting feeling of not being well reduces motivation and thus increases the handicap. The personnel who use cancer rehabilitation techniques should attempt to break and reverse this cycle. Because the cycle involves physical, psychologic, and social aspects, this is best accomplished by a team effort. A team not only is multidisciplinary but also is interdisciplinary. It is a cohesive group. The proper functioning of this group is pivotal to cancer rehabilitation (4).

Setting Up the Cancer Rehabilitation Team

Most medical institutions have physical therapists, occupational therapists, social workers, dietitians, chaplains, and nurses. And they often have a psychologist. The problem has been that all of these professionals, once having been consulted by the primary physician, tend to work in a compartmentalized fashion. Making them part of a team adds to the efficiency and the effectiveness of the entire process.

Specialists in physical medicine and rehabilitation (physiatrists) are trained to be part of such a team. However, if no physiatrist is available, the orthopedic surgeon may have to assume the leadership role. This responsibility is time-consuming. The initial step is the creation of the core group of this cancer rehabilitation team (Table 17-1). This group does the day-to-day rehabilitation. However, other professionals—the extended group—may be needed from time to time (Table 17-1).

How the Team Works

In a large cancer rehabilitation program, separate teams related to orthopedics, oncology, neurology, and so forth can be available. Some key members of the core group, such as the physiatrist, coordinator, and psychologist, are common to all groups, but the allied health professionals who have daily, prolonged contact with the patients, such as the physical and occupational therapists and the social worker, may be different for the different groups.

Referral. The primary service—the orthopedic surgeon—requests consultation by the cancer rehabilitation team. The physiatrist then evaluates the patient, considers the rehabilitation potential, and refers the patient to the appropriate team members, while at the same time informing the coordinator of the new patient. The physiatrist also devises a plan of action and records it on the hospital chart, giving the orthopedic surgeon an opportunity to evaluate the complete plan.

With the referral, a series of interactions occurs (Fig. 17-3). All of this takes place within the time the patient would be hospitalized, whether for surgery, pain management, chemotherapy, or radiation therapy. The rehabilitation program does

Table 17-1. Cancer Rehabilitation Teams

Core group
  Physiatrist
  Psychologist
  Coordinator
  Physical therapist
  Occupational therapist
  Dietitian
  Social worker
  Chaplain
  Nurse
  Orthopedic surgeon
Extended group
  Prosthetist
  Patient visitor (another patient)
  Outside health agency personnel
  Speech pathologist
  Enterostomal therapist
  Vocational counselor

not delay the patient's dismissal if the patient has been seen by the team at admission.

Functions of Various Team Members. Physiatrist. If a physiatrist is not available, another physician interested in the rehabilitative aspects of care should assume responsibility. This physician evaluates the patient and not only delineates the impairment, disability, and handicap but also has knowledge of the psychologic and social aspects of the problem. Knowing the medical problems, this physician guides all of the other allied health professionals and the other physicians involved in the case. He must be able to converse with the patient as well as with the patient's family. He should give encouragement and inspiration to the whole team. The team needs to depend on one member. If agreeable to the surgeon, the physiatrist should be in contact with the patient's family physician in order to inform him of the rehabilitative techniques being used. This member sends reports of the patient's equipment needs, reports to organizations, and reports to the department of vocational rehabilitation.

Coordinator. The professional best trained for this position is a rehabilitation counselor, particularly one who subspecializes in cancer. However, other professionals can assume this role—for example, a registered nurse with an oncology or psychiatric background will be satisfactory for this role. The coordinator ensures that all members of the team communicate, arranges team meetings, helps in the counseling, and provides for the smooth transition between the hospital and the home program.

Psychologist. The primary duty of the psychologist is to arrange for counseling programs. The counseling may be done by a nurse, social worker, or chaplain. In difficult cases, the psychologist assumes the primary responsibility and may recommend consultation with a psychiatrist.

Social Worker. The social worker is vital not only to the financial aspects and the securing of equipment but also to many other aspects of the counseling.

Nurse. The nurse, being most closely associated with the hospitalized patient and the family, is the most obvious member to do basic counseling, to begin the dismissal planning, and to provide for the many physical needs of the patient, such as skin care and bowel and bladder management. The nurse also teaches the activities of daily living.

Chaplain. The chaplain is the one member of the team who is trained to give spiritual counseling, which is usually vital to the patient with cancer.

Physical Therapist. The physical therapist often is most helpful in dealing with the patient's psychologic problems by providing strength, teaching mobility, and supplying equipment, whether it be a prosthesis or a wheelchair. The patient has much rapport with the therapist and can be influenced by the therapist's opinions. The therapist, being aware of the patient's main problem, as well as of other problems through team conferences, usually is able to provide reassurance to the patient more convincingly than other team members.

Occupational Therapist. The occupational therapist has a role similar to that of the physical therapist, although primarily working with upper extremity amputees. The occupational therapist teaches the patient the activities of daily living and helps the patient understand his impairment. Physicians need to encourage the patient to use occupational therapy because such help should make the patient function better.

Dietitian. The dietitian helps in the nutrition of the patient and provides ideas for balancing the diet and for helping the patient overcome the nausea and anorexia that may be attendant to treatment.

Team Conferences. The team conference is the heart of the rehabilitative strategy for the patient. At these conferences, the surgical and adjuvant therapies are intermeshed with the physical plans, the psychologic hurdles, and the social and spiritual predicaments (Table 17-2). Also, this is where the communication occurs, the problems are discussed openly, and the goals are realistically set.

The patient probably should not attend the initial conference. The patient and family, as well as members of the patient's home health agencies, should join later conferences. The patient-care conferences are conducted by the coordinator, but the primary physician and the physiatrist also should be present. Each member brings certain aspects of the patient's care to the conference (Fig. 17-4).

In addition to attending the weekly patient-care conferences, the key team members should meet daily to ensure that new patients are added to the program and that acute problems of the others are discussed. The secretary should provide a list of patients on a daily basis and should distribute this list to all of the team members. Not all team members are needed for all patients at any one time, but they should know which patients are being seen by the team.

Patient Education. The timing of the patient's education should be individualized. Often it is useless to educate the patient about a prosthesis before the amputation. A patient is not as attentive before amputation as he is after. However, a day or two after surgery, the showing of a movie (5) that describes the manufacturing and fitting of the prosthesis and its usefulness

Table 17-2. Discussion at Team Conferences

1. Communication—physical, psychosocial, and spiritual
2. Setting of goals
3. Planning for dismissal—health service needs and equipment needs

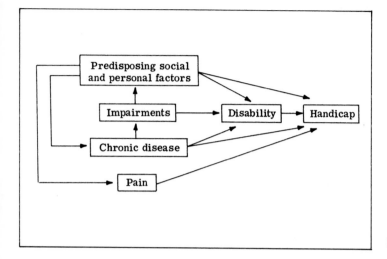

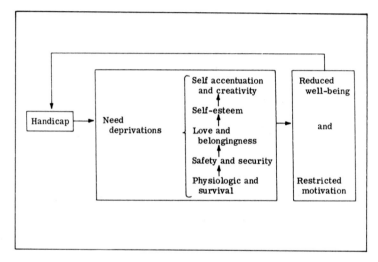

Fig. 17-1. The anatomy of a handicap.

Fig. 17-2. Self-perpetuation of a handicap.

is helpful to both the patient and family. There are also other
movies on the psychologic aspects of amputation.

Patient Visitor. The most effective means of satisfying the
patient's many questions is to have a pool of patient visitors
available. This is particularly important to amputees (6). Amputee visitors are persons who have had amputations. There
should be at least one visitor available with each type of amputation—below-knee, above-knee, hip disarticulation, or hemipelvectomy. The amputee visitors should be of both sexes and
should be screened for suitability, after which they are trained

Rehabilitation

for that role. The amputee visitor is notified after the surgery and is given the name and hospital room number of the patient.

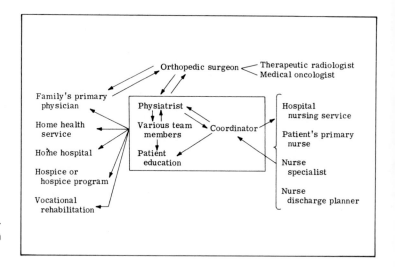

Fig. 17-3. Interaction of cancer rehabilitation team (in box) with other health professionals.

Fig. 17-4. Members participating at a team conference, with their contributions.

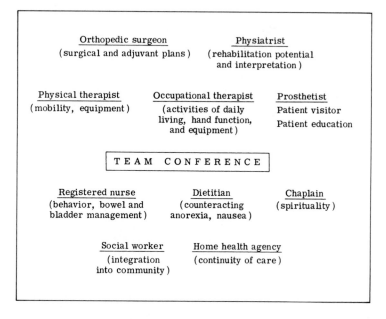

The visitor, 2 days later, contacts the patient, usually by telephone, and asks whether he would like to be visited. Usually there is an obvious change in the patient's attitude once this has been done.

Integration Into the Community. The main goal of the rehabilitative process, both the physical and psychologic aspects, is for the patient to adapt to the disease and impairments and to achieve a realistic independence back within the home community by referral to the home health agency. If a rehabilitation counselor was involved, this counselor should continue the coordinating process. This process may involve domiciliary care, a hospice or hospice program, a nursing home, or a community hospital. More often, however, the need is for vocational rehabilitation and job placement as well as in helping the patient adapt to previous vocational and educational goals.

Apart from the vocational aspects, the very important avocational aspects should be facilitated as much as possible. Amputees should be encouraged to participate in sports. There are handicap ski groups available now, and swimming prostheses also are available (7). Also, the patient and family should be encouraged to attend home group programs. Such a program is "I Can Cope" (8).

If dismissal planning is done carefully while the patient is hospitalized, much time can be saved, and the process of living will continue with as little disturbance as possible. The ultimate proof of effectiveness of the team program is whether the patient and family have learned to cope as a result of the team's efforts.

Some Specific Problems

The Prosthesis. Excellent prosthetic management of an amputee is crucial if rehabilitation is to succeed. Generally, the amputee will require a prosthesis, and life expectancy should not be the only consideration in this decision.

With above-knee and below-knee amputations, the process begins with an immediate postsurgical fitting. Usually, the rigid dressing is changed before the final prosthesis is made. In the past, a rigid plaster-of-paris dressing was used which needed to be changed about three times before the stump had finally shrunk to its smallest size. It is now possible, usually at the time of the second change, when the incision has healed, to manufacture a molded polypropylene temporary socket. This has two components held together with Velcro and has the advantage that the patient can change the size of the socket and thus avoid extra trips to the hospital. In addition, the patient can take off the socket for bathing. If, in addition, the prosthetist provides foam around the pylon, this temporary prosthesis becomes much more cosmetically acceptable. This may be vital to the patient at a time when he is so psychologically vulnerable. It usually requires 6 to 8 weeks before the stump is ready and the final prosthesis can be manufactured. At that time, a careful prescription needs to be made in choosing the most suitable components for the patient's age and intended use. A special prosthesis for use in sports may be recommended (7).

The same principles are employed in the planning of prostheses used after above- or below-elbow amputation as in those used after upper-extremity amputation. A patient with a forequarter amputation should be given a shoulder orthosis as soon as possible. The orthosis is molded of "orthoplast," using the other shoulder as a model, and it can be easily adjusted when the tissue shrinks. The use of this orthosis enables the patient to wear ordinary clothes and retains the patient's shoulder contour. Generally, this is a cosmetic prosthesis rather than a functional one.

Recently, a different method for managing patients with hip disarticulation and hemipelvectomies has been described (9). This new method involves the manufacture of a temporary prosthesis as soon as possible after surgery. The prosthesis is made of lightweight plastic and is molded directly onto the patient. A plastic tubular extension is attached to the socket and is connected to a rubber foot. The second phase of the procedure—the making of the final prosthesis—involves the adaptation of a hydrapneumatic cylinder to an Otto Bock modular system in order to coordinate hip-knee movement in a synergistic way. This overcomes the limitation of having only one cadence with a regular hemipelvectomy prosthesis. Because it is virtually impossible to provide a cable system for forequarter amputations, one group (9) has used myoelectric control of the hand for these patients.

Other Orthopedic Problems. Endoprostheses. Many patients who have undergone amputations have the limb preserved by custom total arthroplasties and endoprostheses. The rehabilitation of these patients requires the same team approach. If this surgical approach is effective, the quality of life will be better sooner, but if a series of operations is needed, these patients often are difficult to rehabilitate.

Fractures. The patient with a pathologic fracture also needs the full team approach. Often such a fracture is the first indication of cancer. The whole rehabilitative protocol is necessary.

Widespread Bony Metastasis. The patient with metastasis needs special rehabilitative measures, particularly if the spinal cord is involved. Modern techniques of bowel and bladder management (such as intermittent catheterization), skin care, teaching of transfers, and proper wheelchair prescriptions can improve the quality of life to the degree that the patient's remaining life can be spent usefully at home. With proper management, life expectancy is often long enough for the patient to be allowed the benefits of a well-trained cancer rehabilitation team.

Hospice. In the United States, the use of hospice programs and hospices is increasing. These help the patient and his family in a number of ways. First, they allow families a respite from the tension produced in caring for such a catastrophically ill person. There is not only a physical but also a psychologic burden on the family unit. Being allowed to have a respite for a week or two revitalizes the family. Second, they help to improve the management of pain. Third, they help the patient cope with and understand the illness. Fourth, they provide a place where the patient can die with dignity.

Long-Term Contractures Due to Treatment. Sometimes even with the eradication and cure of the tumor by excision, with or without an endoprosthesis, muscles are absent and contractures due to scar tissue occur. This may result in a weak limb with pronounced loss of range of motion and may leave the patient with considerable impairment and handicap. A prolonged and well-planned program of physical therapy may help mobilize the limb and make it more functional. Such a program should be started as soon as possible in order to prevent hardening of the scar tissue. The patient must be taught a home program because daily stretching, mobilizing, and strengthening exercises need to be done for months or years. Many of these patients also need an ankle-foot orthosis, such as a posterior leafspring, if there is footdrop due to involvement of the peroneal nerve.

Pain Management. The team approach assists with the management of pain because it helps the patient understand the problems. Bone pain, particularly when associated with fractures and nerve involvement, such as plexopathy, can be very severe. The inadequate use of analgesics for these patients is inexcusable, and the possibility of addiction need not be considered. Most of these patients do not become addicted. The key to management is not to use the analgesics as needed, because once pain is allowed to become severe, it is very difficult to control. However, a round-the-clock schedule of the analgesic often allows the dosage to be reduced (10). With proper management of pain, the patient may revert to his previous character. Multiple drugs usually are not needed. If simpler drugs such as aspirin or codeine are not effective on a 4 hourly schedule, methadone, levorphanol, or morphine should be used. Meperidine is a short-acting drug and usually is of little use. The medication should not interfere with the patient's cognitive abilities. Usually, tranquilizers and antidepressants are unnecessary. If the pain does not respond to oral opioid analgesics, the parenteral route must be used, also on a round-the-clock schedule. Occasionally, a morphine intravenous drip needs to be used. At times, various types of blocks are necessary. The response to transcutaneous electrical nerve stimulation usually is disappointing, but it occasionally helps the patient who has plexopathy or radiculopathy. It is important that one does not experiment with unproved methods but uses a strong analgesic on a regular schedule, as is necessary. There is no harm in dismissing a patient to his home or even to work if there is a well-planned schedule of pain management.

The Pediatric Patient. Some of the long-term effects of cancer treatment in pediatric patients have been well described by Koocher and O'Malley (11). There are special problems with children, not only because of age but also because of the effect on the parents. The effect of amputation, as well as loss of hair and other side effects of the therapy, and the effect on body image may result in long-term psychologic problems, changes in self-esteem, and anxiety. The continuous doubt regarding survival may have consequences not only on the child but also on the family. However, most survivors adjust well to their impairments, and they participate actively in school as well as in social functions. Many lead productive adult lives. They marry and have children, and the quality of their lives may be comparable to that of the rest of the population. However, not all long-term survivors are so fortunate. The rehabilitative team program may prevent poor long-term rehabilitative results.

Documentation and Quantitation.

The proof of the difference a rehabilitative program makes is in the quality of life. This is difficult to measure, and most scales that do are time-consuming and impractical. Recently, Spitzer et al devised a simple, reliable, and valid quality-of-life index that can be completed in a short time and gives profiles of five important areas of living (Table 17-3).

Conclusions

The question is often asked about the rehabilitation potential of an individual patient. If one considers only the grade and stage of the disease, the chance of cure may be good, and consequently the rehabilitation potential should be good. However, if the patient's psychosocial or even physical aspects are not dealt with adequately, the surgeon may well record an excellent result, but the patient and family would think otherwise. The patient's rehabilitation potential was not achieved because the quality of life was such that the cure was not worthwhile to the patient. However, every cancer patient has a rehabilitation potential. The dying patient, for whom nothing can be done—no surgery, chemotherapy, or radiation therapy—has potential to have the quality of life during his last days improved. The pain can be controlled, and provisions can be made for the patient to die with dignity. The anger, frustrations, fears, and anxieties of the patient and the patient's family disappear—to be replaced by satisfaction, self-esteem, and even creativity and

Table 17-3. Quality of Life Index (Score each heading 2, 1, or 0 according to your most recent assessment of the patient)

Activity	*During the last week, the patient:*	
	has been working or studying full-time, or nearly so, in usual occupation; or managing own household; or participating in unpaid or voluntary activities, whether retired or not...	2 ___
	has been working or studying in usual occupation or managing own household or participating in unpaid or voluntary activities; but requiring major assistance or a significant reduction in hours worked or a sheltered situation or was on sick leave	1 ___
	has not been working or studying in any capacity and not managing own household ...	0 ___
Daily living	*During the last week, the patient:*	
	has been self-reliant in eating, washing, toiletting and dressing; using public transport or driving own car...	2 ___
	has been requiring assistance (another person or special equipment) for daily activities and transport but performing light tasks	1 ___
	has not been managing personal care nor light tasks and/or not leaving own home or institution at all...	0 ___
Health	*During the last week, the patient:*	
	has been appearing to feel well or reporting feeling "great" most of the time	2 ___
	has been lacking energy or not feeling entirely "up to par" more than just occasionally	1 ___
	has been very ill or "lousy," seeming weak and washed out most of the time or was unconscious	0 ___
Support	*During the last week:*	
	the patient has been having good relationships with others and receiving strong support from *at least one* family member and/or friend...................................	2 ___
	support received or perceived has been limited from family and friends and/or by the patient's condition	1 ___
	support from family and friends occurred infrequently or only when absolutely necessary or patient was unconscious..	0 ___
Outlook	*During the last week, the patient:*	
	has usually been appearing calm and positive in outlook, accepting and in control of personal circumstances, including surroundings	2 ___
	has sometimes been troubled because not fully in control of personal circumstances or has been having periods of obvious anxiety or depression..........................	1 ___
	has been seriously confused or very frightened or consistently anxious and depressed or unconscious	0 ___
	QL Index Total: ___	

From Spitzer WO, Dobson AJ, Hall J, et al: Measuring the quality of life of cancer patients: a concise QL-Index for use by physicians. J Chronic Dis 34:585–597, 1981. By permission of Pergamon Press.

love. Assurances can be made that the family members will not have feelings of guilt by allowing them to do as much as they can and by allowing them to express their grief without interference. The family members, including young children, need the experience of seeing their loved one lose his body functions as well as die, and they need to accept this. For the health care providers to accomplish all aspects of health care, the surgeon should be part of the whole team. This team can then work together to give the quality of care that fulfills the perceived needs of the patient and family.

References

1. Kostuik JP, Gillespie R (eds): Amputation Surgery and Rehabilitation: the Toronto Experience. New York, Churchill Livingstone, 1981

2. World Health Organization: International Classification of Impairments, Disabilities, and Handicaps: A Manual of Classification Relating to the Consequences of Disease. Geneva, 1980
3. Maslow AH: Motivation and Personality. Second edition. New York, Harper & Row, Publishers, 1970
4. Harvey RF, Jellinek HM, Habeck RV: Cancer rehabilitation: an analysis of 36 program approaches. JAMA 247:2127–2131, 1982
5. McPhee MC, Tryggestad R, Holkestad WL: Road to Recovery (motion picture—1 reel, 30 minutes long, with sound and color, 16 mm). Rochester, Minnesota, Photographic-Audio-visual, Mayo Clinic, 1976
6. May CH, McPhee MC, Pritchard DJ: An amputee visitor program as an adjunct to rehabilitation of the lower limb amputee. Mayo Clin Proc 54:774–778, 1979
7. Kegel B, Webster JC, Burgess EM: Recreational activities of lower extremity amputees: a survey. Arch Phys Med Rehabil 61:258–264, 1980
8. Johnson J: The Effects of a patient education course on persons with a chronic illness. Cancer Nursing 5:117–123, 1982
9. Lehneis HR, project director: Advanced Prosthetics/Orthotics in Cancer Management. Rehabilitation Monograph 63. New York University Medical Center, 1981
10. Lewis BJ: The use of opiate analgesics in cancer patients. Cancer Treat Rep 63:341–342, 1979
11. Koocher GP, O'Malley JE: The Damocles Syndrome: Psychosocial Consequences of Surviving Childhood Cancer. New York, McGraw-Hill Book Company, 1981

INDEX